Magnetic Resonance Imaging

Principles and Applications

This book is dedicated to
Moira, Paul and Laura
and
Barbara, Andrew and Jennifer

Magnetic Resonance Imaging

Principles and Applications

D. M. Kean M.B., Ch.B., D.M.R.D., F.R.C.R.,
Senior Research Fellow and Honorary Consultant,
Department of Medical Radiology,
University of Edinburgh,
Royal Infirmary,
Edinburgh

M. A. Smith B.Sc., M.Sc., Ph.D.,
Principal Physicist and Honorary Fellow,
Department of Medical Physics and Medical Engineering
and Department of Medical Radiology,
University of Edinburgh,
Royal Infirmary,
Edinburgh

SANS TACHE
WILLIAMS & WILKINS
Baltimore

First published in 1986 by
William Heinemann Medical Books
23 Bedford Square, London WC1B 3HH

Library of Congress Cataloging in Publication Data
Kean, D. M.
Magnetic resonance imaging.
1. Magnetic resonance imaging. I. Title
RC 78.7N83K43 1986 616.07'5 85-29617
ISBN 0-683-04554-7

Distributed in North, Central, and South America
by Williams & Wilkins by arrangement with
William Heinemann Medical Books

Printed in Great Britain

Contents

Acknowledgements

We are extremely grateful to the following for supplying us with many of the images which appear in the book: Dr. Graeme Bydder, Hammersmith Hospital, London (Picker superconducting system), Dr. Michael Modic, Cleveland Clinic, Cleveland (Technicare superconducting system), Dr. Hedvig Hricak, UCSF, San Francisco (Diasonics superconducting system) and Prof. B. S. Worthington, Queens Medical Centre, Nottingham (prototype Picker resistive system). The remaining images are from the Edinburgh NMR Imaging Unit (M & D resistive system) which is funded by the Medical Research Council, Scottish Home and Health Department, Lothian Health Board, University of Edinburgh, Melville Trust and Wellcome Trust.

We would particularly like to thank Prof. Jonathan Best for his advice and encouragement during the preparation of the book. We are also indebted to Dr. Peter Tothill and Dr. Paul Allan for their valuable comments on the manuscript. Finally we wish to acknowledge Mrs Colette Rowan for secretarial services, Mrs Joan Smith for proof reading and Miss Ruth Douglas for radiographic services.

Foreword

The introduction of magnetic resonance into the sphere of clinical medicine has created an exciting opportunity for diagnosticians and basic scientists involved in imaging techniques. The application of an *in vitro* chemical technique for the *in vivo* analysis of living tissues will impact heavily on to the delivery of health care.

The advent of any clinically oriented technology creates an information gap concerning its physical basis and applicability, and, magnetic resonance (MR) is clearly different. It has no ionizing radiation, and its imaging principles are also different than those now in use. Therefore, new perceptions are called for, and the imager must now think in terms of subatomic interactions of the nucleus rather than of the electron which forms the basis of conventional radiography. Information can now be obtained which depends on a complex interaction of various parameters potentially allowing tissue characterization in both the normal and diseased states. The MR signal provides not only morphological data but biochemical data as well. This knowledge should lead to a more fundamental understanding of the natural history of disease and its response to therapy.

The potential of MR as a cross-sectional imaging device is already obvious and has spawned hundreds of papers documenting its use in a variety of clinical situations. As awareness of this technique grows, a need for a more fundamental understanding of its multidisciplinary nature emerges in order that the imager might become a more informed user. There will continue to be an ongoing exchange between the basic research scientists who develop, and the clinical imager who applies. As in any other rapidly evolving field, there will be controversies which are resolved, as well as information which will become outdated before texts or even scientific journals make their way into press.

Nevertheless, the need still exists for basic texts such as this which provide an introduction of the background, techniques, applicability and limitations of magnetic resonance imaging (MRI) and which will not intimidate the newcomer. The early chapters of this text provide an historical background and an explanation of basic MR physics. This is followed by a summary of the types of equipment, techniques, instrumentation and the imaging process. Possible biological effects and concerns are also reviewed. Finally, the clinical potential of MRI, which correlates and develops upon its basic science and physical considerations, is discussed.

This book is not meant as an encyclopedic reference work, but it is a concise, well-written, thoroughly understandable text which should be of great value to the medical student, house officer or clinician seeking an introduction to this fast-moving and exciting new technology.

Michael T. Modic, 1986
Director, Divisions of Neuroradiology and Magnetic Resonance Imaging. University Hospitals of Cleveland, Ohio.

I

Introduction

Early history

The application of nuclear magnetic resonance (NMR) in the field of medicine has been hailed as a major innovation. Though NMR is relatively new to the field of medicine the technique itself has been around for nearly 40 years. The phenomenon was first discovered in 1946 by Bloch and Purcell, two researchers who were working independently, for which they were awarded the Nobel Prize in 1952.

During the next 25 years NMR developed into a widely used technique for non-destructive analysis of small samples. In particular NMR spectroscopy became a major analytical tool, being able to identify the various different chemical states of elements whose properties made them suitable candidates for NMR analysis. Such spectral analysis required very uniform magnetic fields often of quite high field strengths. The technological difficulties of constructing such magnets meant that the samples which could be investigated were small, of the order of millimetres in size. Many of the applications of NMR in the 1950s and 1960s were concerned with investigations at the microscopic level. More recently NMR has been applied at a more macroscopic level, in particular by the food industry in the investigation of water content or what is sometimes referred to as the mobile proton content.

Two factors were primarily responsible for the decision in various research centres and commercial companies to investigate the possibility of developing a technique of NMR imaging *in vivo*. The first one was the work of Damadian (1971) who demonstrated that a particular NMR parameter (T_1) of tumour samples, measured *in vitro*, was significantly higher than normal tissues. This exciting finding kindled many people's imagination, all of whom came to the same conclusion: a technique which could differentiate between tissues of different pathological types would have potentially immense diagnostic potential if *in vivo* images in the human body could be obtained. The second factor which stimulated the interest in the development of NMR imaging is more indirect. This was the impact of X-ray computerised tomography (CT) on medical imaging. Computerised tomography presented images in a way that was completely new to many clinicians. It demonstrated the advantages of imaging a patient by tomographic sections through the head or body. The impact of CT was so great, and CT installations proliferated so fast, that the United States introduced legislation to limit the number of CT units within a given region.

There are three areas in which CT motivated research centres and commercial companies to develop NMR imaging. The first is that the medical world became used to viewing the body in tomographic sections and recognised the value of such techniques. Secondly CT opened the door to high cost, high technology medical imaging. Lastly it demonstrated the commercial rewards available for a comparable imaging technique such as NMR imaging. From the start it became clear that NMR imaging was going to be 'big business'.

There is a fair amount of contention as to who exactly is the 'father of NMR imaging'. This honour is claimed, with varying degrees of assertion, by a number of people. In fact there were a number of groups, both in the United States and in Great Britain, who were simultaneously investigating different methods of NMR imaging. This book, which is intended to be an introduction to the subject, is not the place to undertake a detailed analysis of the various claims. However there are three publications that had a considerable impact on the subject. The first (Damadian, 1971) has already been mentioned. The second was the first published paper which discussed and presented results of NMR imaging; this was a paper by Lauterbur (1973) who used linear magnetic field gradients to obtain spatial information and the technique of back projection reconstruction, as used in CT, to obtain an image. The third publication which had a major influence was that relating to the use of a two-dimensional Fourier transform technique for image production which was published by the Aberdeen group (Edelstein *et al.*, 1980). Two-dimensional Fourier transform as a method of image production was demonstrated to be superior to other image reconstruction techniques and has been almost universally adopted in present-day NMR imaging systems.

Terminology

As various techniques of NMR imaging were developed so the terms used to describe the basic technique proliferated. Zeugmatography was proposed fairly early on by Lauterbur and was derived from the Greek word zeugma, meaning yoke. The rationale behind this was that NMR imaging essentially involved the 'yoking together' of magnetism and radiofrequency (RF) radiation. As might have been predicted this rather contrived term never really caught on. Alternative terms to NMR imaging that have been proposed are: spin imaging, spin mapping or NMR tomography. More recently the term magnetic resonance imaging (MRI) has become widely accepted as an alternative to the term NMR imaging. MRI is favoured in general by clinicians who are using the technique, the rationale being that the word nuclear could have unfavourable connotations in the mind of the general public. As many NMR imagers would be sited in specially built installations it is suggested that the presence of the word nuclear would cause unnecessary concern. It is fair to say that most clinicians now favour the use of the term MRI, although those physicists, engineers and scientists working on the development of the technique still generally refer to it as NMR imaging. As this book is designed as an introduction primarily to clinicians not familiar with the field of NMR the term MRI will be used where appropriate.

Principles of NMR and MRI

This book is intended as an introduction to both the physical principles and clinical applications of MRI. The physical principles of NMR are quite different from other techniques in diagnostic radiology and consequently require some explanation. The principles of NMR described in Chapter 2 are common to both MRI and NMR spectroscopy. It has been mentioned already that NMR was initially used for spectroscopic analysis and it is important to stress again the fact that MRI and NMR spectroscopy are quite separate techniques even though the fundamental principles are common to both. The majority of MRI systems in use at present are incapable of doing spectroscopy, the exceptions being some of the high field systems which are being installed. This book concentrates on the imaging aspects of NMR; an introduction to the use of NMR spectroscopy for *in vivo* analysis, or topical magnetic resonance (TMR) as it is sometimes called, can be found elsewhere (Gadian, 1982).

The view is sometimes expressed that it is not necessary to understand the principles of NMR in order to use an MRI system. However, one aspect of MRI that is different from other imaging techniques is that there are three variables in an NMR image—proton density, T_1 and T_2—compared with a single variable in almost all other imaging techniques. As a consequence the method of imaging will dramatically alter the contrast, or film density if the image is displayed on transparent film, between different tissues in the image. The aspect of MRI which influences the contrast between tissues in the image is the pulse sequence used. Chapter 3 is devoted to this aspect of MRI but it will be apparent that to use MRI to its full potential, some understanding of the principles of NMR is essential. Unfortunately to obtain the same response the timing of pulse sequences in MRI is different for systems with different field strengths so it is not possible to recommend pulse sequences that are universally applicable.

The principles behind image formation are described in Chapter 4. Some imaging techniques such as steady state free precession (SSFP) and field focused nuclear magnetic resonance (FONAR) were developed in the early days of MRI but have been discarded in favour of more efficient or more clinically useful methods. These methods, though of historical interest, will not be described as they are not relevant for the understanding of present-day MRI. A more detailed explanation of some of the principles and technical aspects of MRI systems can be found elsewhere (Mansfield and Morris, 1982).

Hardware

The hardware that is used in MRI equipment is described in Chapter 5. The technology associated with magnetism and radiofrequency radiation was unfamiliar to many research centres and commercial companies. That and the complexity of MRI systems probably account for the relatively long interval between the first crude NMR images and commercially available systems, approximately 10 years for MRI compared with about 3 years for X-ray CT. The various components are described as are the various factors to consider when installing such a system.

Clinical applications of MRI

The clinical applications of MRI are described in the remaining chapters, each chapter dealing with a separate part of the body. MRI is still being evaluated and its precise role in clinical practice is still to be defined. However, even at this early stage in its development certain important points can be made. MRI is the modality of choice in the investigation of the central nervous system and spine. It is at least equal to the other modalities in the liver, pancreas and the retroperitoneum. It appears to have the potential to be superior in the pelvis and some parts of the musculoskeletal system, for example, bony neoplasms. The aim of the clinical section of this book is therefore to outline the applications of MRI, to highlight the advantages without omitting the disadvantages, and where possible to give some guidance regarding the most appropriate MRI technique to employ and to suggest areas where improvements may be expected in the future. It is realised that some suggestions may turn out to be wrong, not necessarily out of ignorance but due to rapid progress and the knowledge that continuing experience brings. An effort has been made to keep personal preferences out of the text, and as can be seen from the illustrations many different types and makes of imager are represented.

Some of the early workers in the field of MRI made rather exaggerated claims as to the technique's potential applications. As a consequence many people's expectations of MRI have been raised to levels which would be impossible to satisfy. A very real fear is that because MRI is unable to live up to some of these rather exalted expectations it may lose credibility. Our aim therefore in this book is to present as balanced a view of MRI as possible, showing not only its advantages but also areas where other techniques are clinically superior.

2

Fundamentals of the NMR experiment

Introduction

In this chapter we will consider how an NMR signal is obtained and describe the various parameters associated with it. The physical principles described are fundamental to all aspects of NMR, whether it is being used for spectroscopic analysis of small samples or imaging of the human body. In both cases the underlying principles behind the signal production are the same. In order to describe the physical principles of NMR it is necessary to use either the classical model of the atom or quantum physics. Both methods of explanation are valid, but experience has shown that a clearer understanding of the NMR experiment, ranging initially from the response of an individual nucleus to finally the signal detected from a sample, is obtained using classical rather than quantum physics. Consequently the former will be used throughout the book.

The term nuclear magnetic resonance gives a good indication of the basis of the technique. It is the nucleus of the atom which is of interest and its ability to resonate under certain conditions in the presence of a magnetic field. Hitherto the physical principles of most aspects of diagnostic radiology had been concerned with interactions with the electron shell of an atom, in particular its ability to produce or attenuate X-rays. The basic stages of the NMR process are illustrated diagrammatically in Fig. 2.1. The sample, in this case a human body, is initially placed in a large magnetic field which remains constant throughout the NMR experiment. Then follow two quite separate stages of the NMR process. The sample is exposed to an oscillating magnetic field in the radiofrequency (RF) region of the electromagnetic spectrum, causing the nuclei in the sample to resonate. This RF radiation is then switched off but the nuclei continue to resonate resulting in the next stage of the NMR experiment which is the emission of the RF radiation from these resonating nuclei which can be detected as an NMR signal. There is therefore something of a philosophical difference between NMR and other radiological techniques. In these latter the body interacts with a beam of X-rays or ultrasound, attenuating or reflecting it respectively. This is not so with NMR; the RF radiation transmitted through

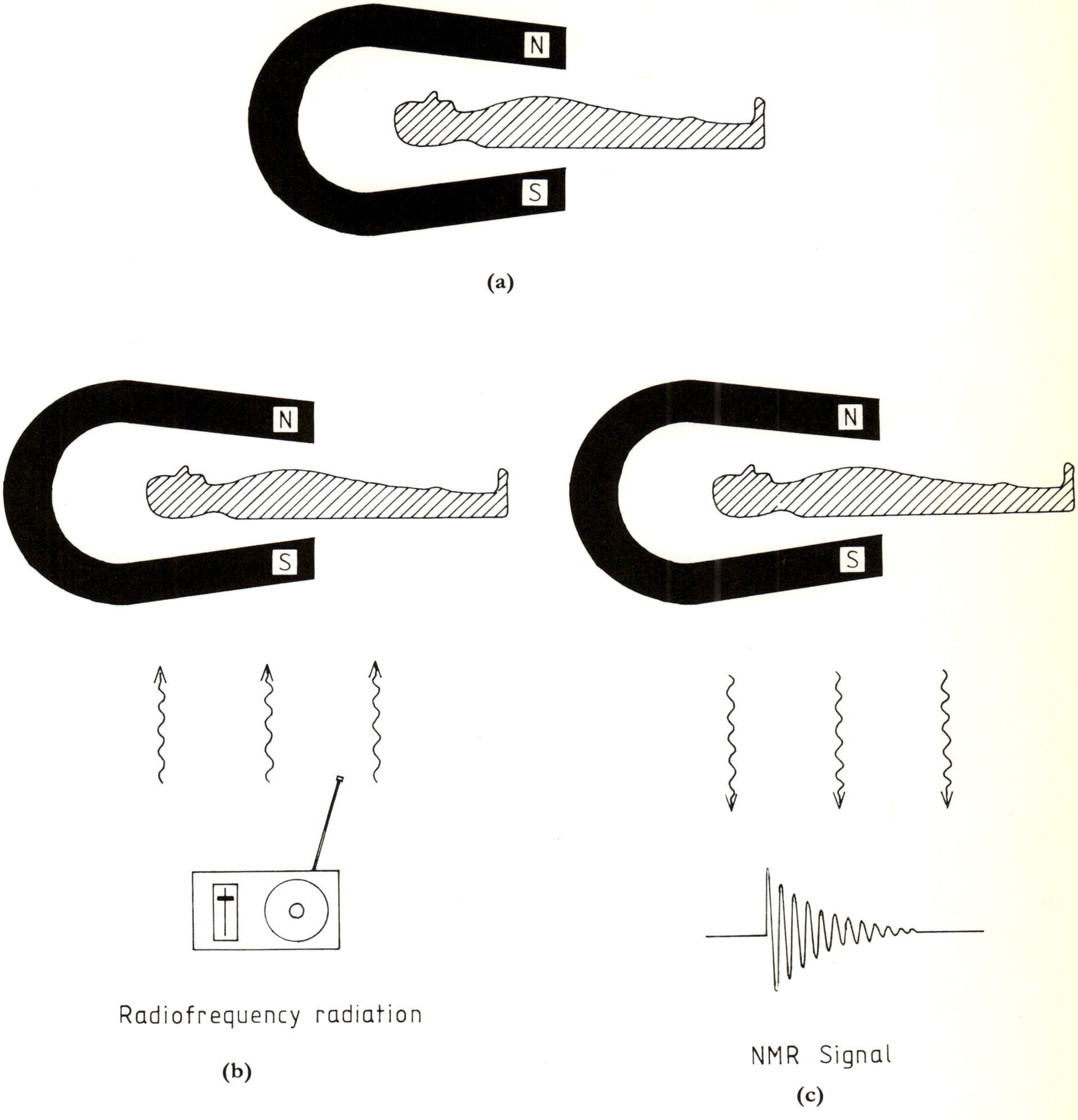

Fig. 2.1 The different stages of NMR. *(a)* A sample, for example a patient, is placed in a strong constant magnetic field *(b)* radiofrequency radiation is then applied to produce resonance within the sample and finally, after the radiofrequency radiation has been switched off *(c)* the emitted radiofrequency radiation from the resonating nuclei is detected, producing the NMR signal

the patient is not being attenuated or reflected, it is stimulating the tissue itself to produce a signal.

Nuclei

The technique of NMR cannot be applied to all nuclei. Only nuclei which are: (*a*) rotating and therefore possessing the property known as spin, and (*b*) possess an odd number of protons and neutrons, can be made to resonate. Such nuclei have an intrinsic magnetism, or magnetic moment, that makes each nucleus a magnetic dipole—in effect, a bar magnet. A useful analogy is to consider a spinning nucleus as the earth which possesses a similar though much larger magnetic moment (Fig. 2.2). Examples of some of the nuclei that can be measured using NMR and of particular interest in medicine are listed in Table 2.1.

The NMR sensitivity refers to the size of the signal which would be obtained from an equal number of nuclei at the same field strength, scaled relative to hydrogen. It can be seen that sensitivity is highest for hydrogen closely followed by fluorine. There is a considerable difference in the amount of the different elements in the human body, and the column labelled 'measurement sensitivity' in Table 2.1 refers to the NMR sensitivity multiplied by the relative numbers of the nuclei within the human body. The measurement sensitivity of hydrogen is now several orders of magnitude greater than the other nuclei. The nucleus which is used for MRI is the hydrogen atom, and because the nucleus of the hydrogen atom con-

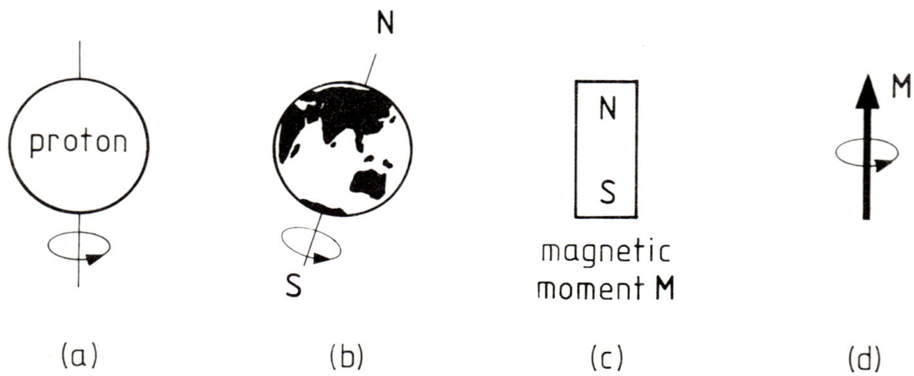

Fig. 2.2 *(a)* The proton can be considered as a sphere which, because of spin, rotates about its axis. *(b)* This is analogous, on a much larger scale, to the earth rotating on its axis with its resultant magnetic field. *(c)* Such a magnetic field from a rotating body can be considered as a bar magnet with a magnetic moment *M*. *(d)* In NMR a single proton is often represented by an arrow pointing in the direction of the magnetic field with a magnetic moment *M*

Table 2.1 Nuclei of interest in biological NMR

Nucleus	*NMR sensitivity*	*Measurement sensitivity*
^{1}H	1	1
^{31}P	6.6×10^{-2}	3.7×10^{-6}
^{23}Na	9.3×10^{-2}	6.0×10^{-5}
^{13}C	1.6×10^{-2}	4.6×10^{-5}
^{19}F	8.3×10^{-1}	2.7×10^{-7}

The relative sensitivity refers to the relative size of the NMR signal, normalised to that obtained from protons, obtained from an equal number of nuclei at a constant field strength. The measurement sensitivity is a combination of the relative sensitivity and the number of the particular nuclei present in the human body; this gives an indication of the size of the NMR signal obtainable for MRI

tains only a single proton the technique of MRI may sometimes be referred to as proton NMR.

Nuclei within a sample are randomly orientated so that the magnetic moments from the individual nuclei effectively cancel each other out and there is no net magnetic moment. However, when the sample is placed in a magnetic field, the nuclei within the sample tend to align themselves with the direction of the external magnetic field, producing a net magnetic moment in the direction of the magnetic field. In fact the nuclei within the sample tend to align themselves parallel and anti-parallel to the direction of the magnetic field, slightly over half having their own magnetic moment in the same direction as the magnetic field. For example 0.4 excess protons will align with the magnetic field per million protons at 0.1 T (see below) and 37°C. The net magnetisation of the sample is therefore very small and is proportional to the magnetic field strength. The magnetic field in which the sample is placed is often referred to as the external magnetic field to avoid confusion with any magnetic field generated within the sample, and is commonly referred to by the symbol H_0. The units of magnetic field are Tesla and Gauss: 1 T (Tesla) = 10000 G (Gauss). The magnitude of the magnetic fields used in NMR can be appreciated by considering the fact that the earth's magnetic field is approximately 0.05 mT (0.5 G).

Precession

Let us now consider an individual nucleus which is aligned in the same direction as the external magnetic field which we will assume is in the vertical or z coordinate direction. This nucleus is represented pictorially in Fig. 2.3(*a*) as a rotating arrow, the direction of the arrow representing the direction of the magnetic moment of the nucleus. If an oscillating magnetic field is now applied in the horizontal plane at the correct frequency the nucleus will resonate. The resonance of the nucleus takes the form of precession about the equilibrium position. The term precession can be understood by considering the vertical arrow which represents the nucleus (Fig. 2.3(*b*)). The base remains fixed while the top describes a circle of gradually increasing radius so that the arrow is at an ever-increasing angle α to the vertical. The frequency of the oscillating magnetic field in the horizontal plane which produces this precession, or resonance, is called the Larmor frequency derived from the following equation:

$$\omega = \gamma H_o$$

where

ω = Larmor frequency

γ = gyromagnetic ratio which is constant for a particular nucleus

H_o = external magnetic field

The frequency of the oscillating magnetic field in the horizontal plane which produces the precession is in the megahertz (1 MHz = 10^6 cycles/s) or radiofrequency (RF) region of the electromagnetic spectrum. For this reason, and because the duration of the oscillating magnetic field is fairly short, it is generally referred to as the RF pulse. The amplitude and duration of the RF pulse will determine the precession angle α—the larger the pulse the larger the angle. As a consequence the RF pulse is named after the size of the precession angle it produces. The magnetic moment of a nucleus at an angle α to the vertical can be represented by its three components, M_z, M_y and M_x. When an RF pulse is applied the horizontal component of the magnetic moment will gradually increase until, in the case of a 90° pulse, it is equal to M. This is illustrated in Fig. 2.4.

The frequency of precession of the nucleus about the vertical axis is also the Larmor frequency. When the nucleus has been tipped through an angle α, which in the case illustrated in Fig. 2.3 is 90°, and the RF pulse is switched off, the nucleus precesses back to its original equilibrium position again at the Larmor frequency. The component of the magnetic moment rotating in the horizontal plane perpendicular to the external magnetic field would induce an electric

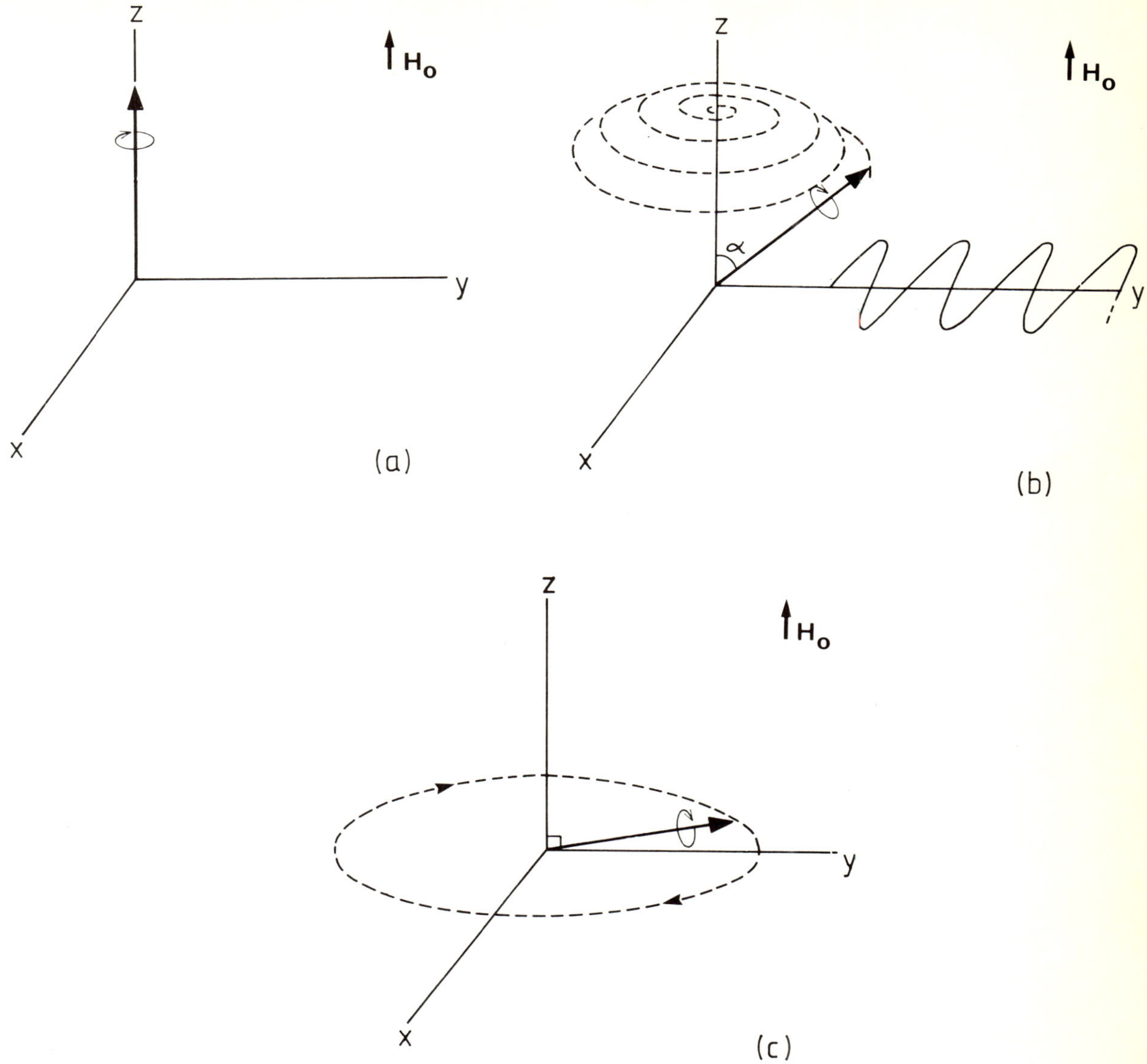

Fig. 2.3 *(a)* A single proton is aligned in the direction of the external magnetic field. *(b)* An oscillating magnetic field in the horizontal plane (an RF pulse at the Larmor frequency) causes the nucleus to precess, the angle α gradually increasing with time. *(c)* With sufficient RF pulse the nucleus can eventually be at 90° to the external magnetic field

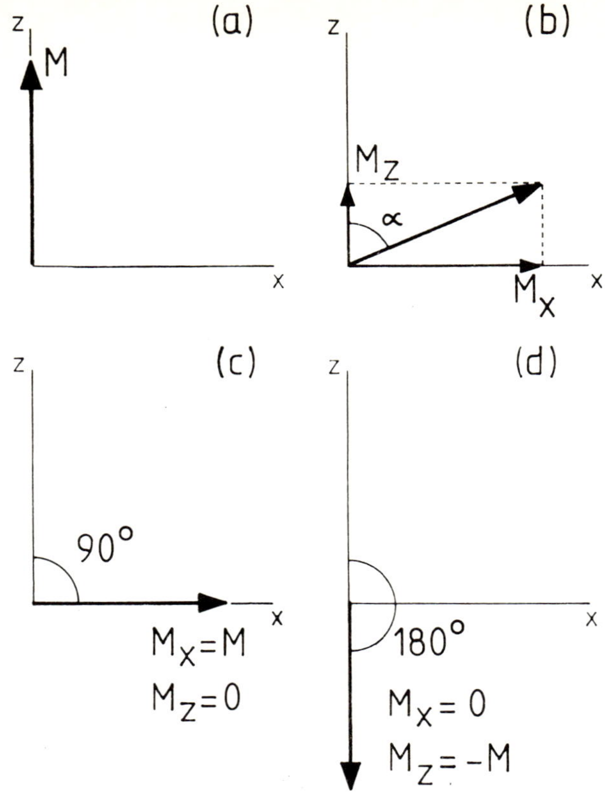

Fig. 2.4 *(a)* The nucleus with magnetic moment M is initially in the z direction when it is at equilibrium. *(b)* Following the application of an RF pulse the nucleus is tipped through angle α; at this angle the magnetic moment M of the nucleus has three components, M_x, M_y and M_z though only two are shown in the illustration. *(c)* If sufficient RF is applied the nucleus is tipped through 90° and the component of magnetisation M_x is equal to M and the component M_z is equal to zero. *(d)* The application of more RF radiation causes the nucleus to precess until it is at 180° to its equilibrium position when the component of magnetisation M_x equals zero and the component M_z equals $-M$

current in a receiver coil round the sample and so an NMR signal would be detected, though in practice a signal cannot be obtained from a single nucleus.

The other type of RF pulse which is often used in NMR is the 180° pulse. Such a pulse will cause the nucleus to precess through the horizontal plane until it is 180° from its original equilibrium position. An example of a 180° pulse is illustrated in Fig. 2.4.

Following a 90° pulse a nucleus rotates in the horizontal plane, its position in the plane being defined by the phase angle ϕ. The phase of the nucleus varies with time as it rotates. Figure 2.5 illustrates a nucleus at slightly different times and therefore different phases.

Of course it is impossible to do any sort of experiment with a single nucleus, so to understand some of the NMR parameters we must consider the more practical situation of a sample containing a large number of nuclei. The sample is placed in a hypothetical perfectly uniform external magnetic field H_0 and a 90° RF pulse is applied. If, as before, we consider the initial equilibrium position to be in the vertical direction then the nuclei all precess through 90° until they are rotating in the horizontal plane. Immediately after the RF pulse all the arrows representing the magnetic moment of each nuclei are pointing in the same direction and they will all be precessing together. The nuclei all have the same phase angle ϕ which is often referred to as 'being in phase' or 'possessing phase coherence'. Because all the individual magnetic moments are pointing in the same direction there will be a large net magnetic moment rotating in the horizontal plane which will produce a signal in an RF receiver coil.

Although the sample containing the nuclei is in a hypothetically perfectly uniform external magnetic field each nucleus within the sample will experience an additional minute magnetic field produced by the magnetic moments of other surrounding precessing nuclei. There are therefore minute variations in the local field throughout the sample causing corresponding minute variations in the Larmor frequency. This results in the nuclei precessing at slightly different frequencies, and so after a short time the nuclei are not all exactly in phase and there is some loss of phase coherence. This process is illustrated in Fig. 2.6 where it can be seen that initially there is a large magnetic moment along the y axis when all the nuclei are in phase. A short time later, because the nuclei precess at slightly different frequencies, they are not all in line and as a consequence the net magnetic moment in the horizontal plane is correspondingly reduced. Remember—it is the component in the horizontal plane which produces the NMR signal. Shortly afterwards the nuclei have precessed more back towards equilibrium, and they have lost even

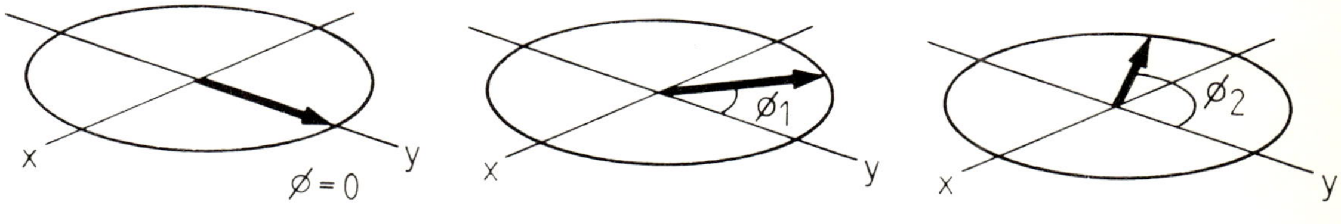

Fig. 2.5 A nucleus at different times following a 90° pulse. The nucleus is rotating in the xy plane and the phase angle ϕ is the angle between the nucleus and one of the horizontal axes

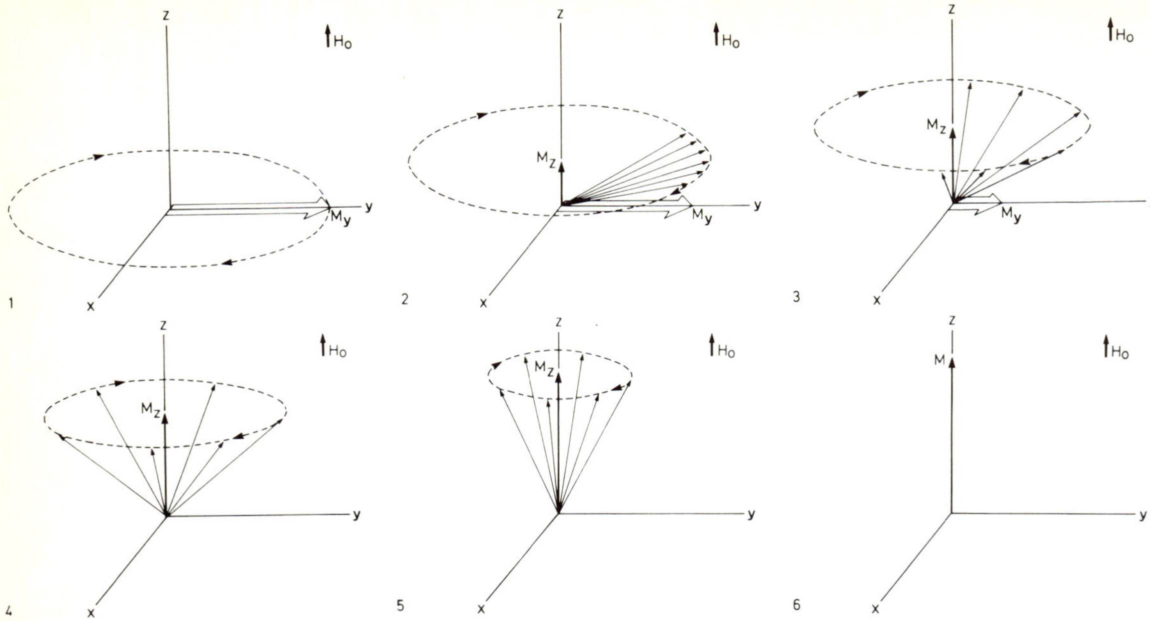

Fig. 2.6 Consider a group of six nuclei within a sample. *(1)* Following a 90° pulse there is a net magnetic moment from the nuclei in the horizontal plane. It is the rotation of this component of the magnetic field which produces the NMR signal which can be detected. *(2)* As the nuclei start precessing back towards equilibrium they gradually lose phase coherence and the component of net magnetisation in the horizontal plane is reduced. *(3)* As time progresses the horizontal component of magnetisation will be reduced further until eventually all the nuclei are out of phase *(4)* and so there is no component of net magnetisation in the horizontal plane. *(5)* The nuclei continue to precess until *(6)* equilibrium is reached

more phase coherence such that the component M_y is now very small. Eventually after a further time interval there is complete loss of phase coherence, and as the horizontal components of the nuclei are randomly arranged there is no component in the horizontal plane and hence no signal is produced. Note in Fig. 2.6 that this occurs before the nuclei have returned to the vertical equilibrium position. The nuclei in the sample continue to precess out of phase until they have all returned to the vertical equilibrium position.

T_1 and T_2

The variation in the net components of magnetic moment with time is shown in Fig. 2.7 illustrating the corresponding positions of the six examples in Fig. 2.6. After the RF pulse the component M_y oscillates and we can see an NMR signal. In this theoretical example with a perfectly uniform magnetic field the envelope of the decay of the NMR signal is an exponential with a time constant which

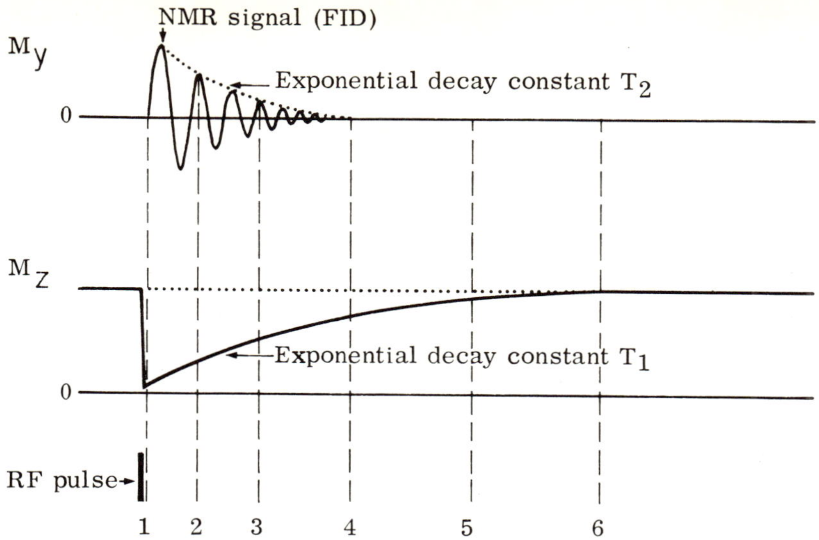

Fig. 2.7 The relationship between the state of the nuclei in Fig. 2.6 and the NMR signal, T_1 and T_2. The numbers 1 to 6 shown at the bottom of the figure refer to the time corresponding to the six diagrams in Fig. 2.6. The envelope of the NMR signal is only T_2 in the hypothetical situation of a perfectly uniform magnetic field

is referred to as the T_2 relaxation time. The decay of the NMR signal is due to the loss of phase coherence, which in turn is due to very small variations in the magnetic field caused by interactions between the precessing or spinning nuclei.

The vertical component of magnetisation M_z drops to zero immediately after the RF pulse and takes longer to return to equilibrium. This return to equilibrium is also an exponential with a decay constant which is referred to as the T_1 relaxation.

In practice it is impossible to get a perfectly uniform magnetic field, and so there are always variations in the magnetic field within a sample in addition to those caused by the spinning nuclei. We saw how variations in the overall magnetic field produced by the minute magnetic fields from surrounding nuclei caused loss of phase coherence and therefore decay of the NMR signal; it follows, therefore, that if the variations in the external magnetic field are too great the loss of phase coherence will occur so quickly that no NMR signal can be detected. For spectroscopic analysis of small samples an external magnetic field uniformity, also referred to as inhomogeneity, of 1 part in 10^7 is required. For imaging purposes an inhomogeneity of 1 in 10^4 to 1 in 10^5 is sufficient. The effect of the variations in the external magnetic field which will always be present causes the NMR signal to decay faster than it would do in the theoretical situation of a perfectly uniform external field considered earlier. The envelope of an NMR signal obtained in practice has a decay constant which is referred to as T_2*. The following is always true:

$$T_2^* \ll T_2 \leq T_1$$

An NMR signal which is detected immediately after an RF pulse is called free induction decay (FID). The term implies that precession occurs in the absence of a driving RF field, and is therefore free. An NMR signal is often referred to as an FID. It is also possible to delay the NMR signal so that an echo is produced (see Chapter 3). Although both signals are theoretically FIDs, a signal which occurs immediately after an RF pulse is generally referred to as an FID, whereas a signal which occurs some time after the RF pulse is called an echo. An example of both types of NMR signal is illustrated in Fig. 2.8.

As the NMR signal is produced by the component of magnetic moment in the horizontal plane, the size of the signal is directly related to the size of this component. Therefore the amplitude of the NMR signal is largest following a 90° pulse and zero following a 180° pulse. The phase of the net component of magnetisation in the horizontal plane also affects the NMR signal as illustrated in Fig. 2.9. An NMR signal, whether an FID or an echo, contains four separate components: amplitude, frequency, phase and duration of resonance, as illustrated in Fig. 2.10. Although the NMR signal possesses four separate components, none of these are the important T_1 or T_2 relaxation times. The initial amplitude of a single NMR signal is a function of the amount of nuclei present, and the duration of resonance (T_2*) is simply a measure of the inhomogeneity of the external magnetic field. It is not possible therefore to measure T_1 or T_2 from a single NMR signal. To obtain such information we must use different types of pulse sequences as described in Chapter 3.

The return to vertical or longitudinal equilibrium following an RF pulse is described by the exponential decay constant T_1 and is due to the transfer of energy from the precessing nuclei to other larger molecules which are not resonating. This interaction between spinning nuclei and the surrounding molecular lattice structure has resulted in the term 'spin-lattice relaxation' which is synonymous with the term T_1 relaxation. The term lattice may suggest something solid though in fact it refers to anything in the environment of the precessing nuclei whether liquid or solid. A further term that is sometimes used to describe this process, equivalent to both T_1 relaxation and spin-lattice relaxation, is 'longitudinal relaxation'.

T_2 relaxation time is the time constant which describes the exponential loss of phase coherence due to very small variations in

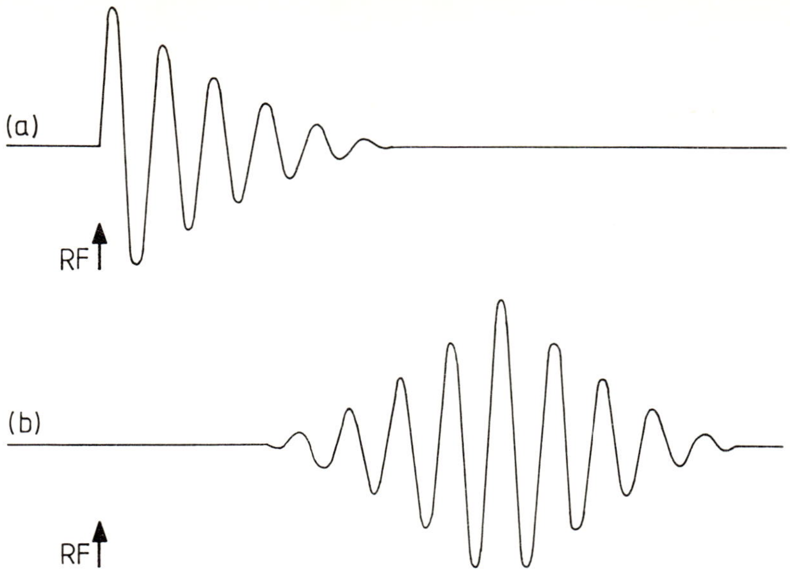

Fig. 2.8 Two types of NMR signals (FID): *(a)* signal detected immediately after an RF pulse, and *(b)* echo detected some time after the RF pulse

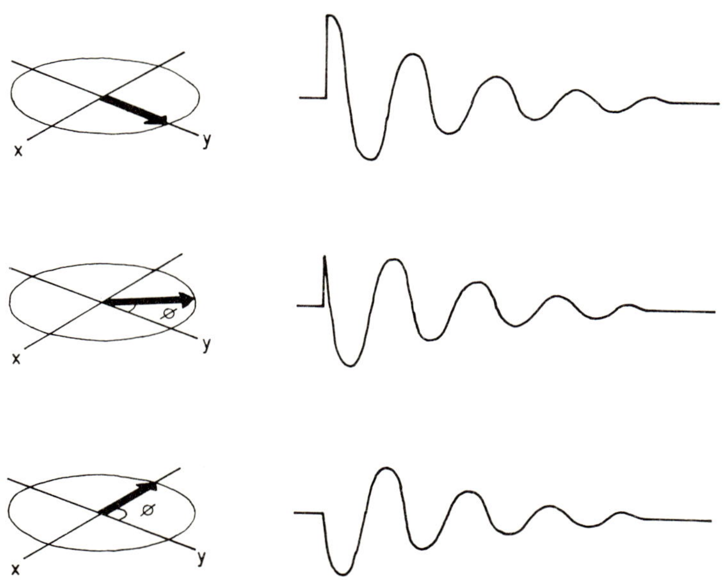

Fig. 2.9 Separate phase angles with their corresponding NMR signals. The NMR signal displayed is a variation of one of the components of magnetisation in the horizontal plane, in this case M_y, with time. When the phase angle ϕ equals zero the signal will initially be large and as the phase angle increases to 90° the starting position of the signal will be reduced. Consequently the position of the peaks of the NMR signal with time is a function of the phase angle

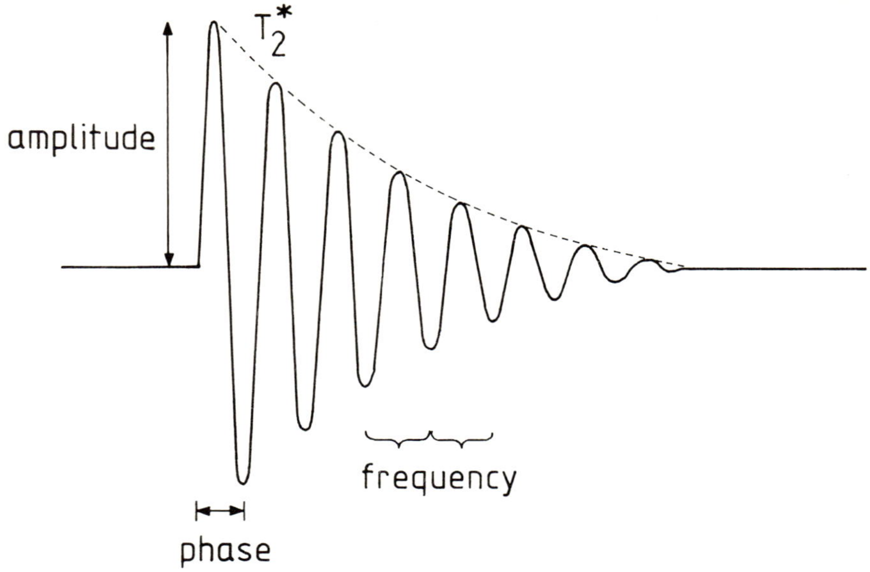

Fig. 2.10 The four components of an NMR signal. In practice the envelope of the NMR signal is not T_2 but T_2* due to inhomogeneities of the external magnetic field which are always present

the magnetic field caused by interactions between the spinning nuclei. The loss of phase coherence occurs in the horizontal or transverse plane and so the two synonymous terms for T_2 relaxation are 'spin-spin relaxation' and 'transverse relaxation'.

Biological T_1 and T_2

Although the NMR signal detected in MRI comes from protons within the body, not all will produce a signal. Protons giving rise to an NMR signal are mainly those in cellular water, which constitutes by far the greatest proportion of protons in the body, and lipids. Those in macromolecules such as proteins, DNA and solid structures such as bone do not usually contribute to the NMR signal. As the majority of any NMR signal will come from water within the tissues, it is the behaviour of this water which largely determines the values of T_1 and T_2 in MRI. The biological mechanisms which influence T_1 and T_2 relaxation times are not yet fully understood, though it is generally accepted that the concept of free and bound water gives the best understanding of T_1 though it may be to some extent an oversimplified model. In tissue a proportion of the water is bound to the surface of proteins and as a consequence its motion is slowed by its proximity to the larger molecules. This results in a lowering of the T_1 value. Other water in the tissue will not be bound to protein and is considered to be free, resulting in it having a higher T_1—T_1 of pure water, equivalent to free water in the tissue, is of the order of 3 s at a field strength of 0.1 T. T_1 in tissue is much lower than this, and will depend on the relative proportions of free and bound water within the tissue—the larger the proportion of free water the higher the T_1, the larger the proportion of bound water the lower the T_1. It is generally assumed that the increase in T_1 in tumour tissue compared with normal tissue is due to a release of bound water into the tissue resulting in an increase in free water.

The effect of frequency on the two relaxation parameters is quite different. As the strength of the magnet used for MRI is increased the resonant frequency will also increase. As the resonant frequency increases so T_1 also increases. It is not therefore possible to quote the T_1 value for a particular tissue without stipulating the frequency at which it was measured. This causes considerable difficulties in comparing *in vivo* tissue measurements on patients using different MRI systems, as often different field strengths are used. Not only will the T_1 values of different tissues increase as the resonant frequency increases, differences between them will steadily be reduced until all the tissue's T_1 tends towards that for pure water. The magnitude of the change in T_1 with frequency can be appreciated by considering T_1 of white matter in the brain which varies from 278 ms at 0.08 T to 500 ms at 0.26 T.

Compared with the large variation in T_1 with frequency there is very little variation in T_2 with frequency, and most biological tissues have a T_2 value in the range of about 50–150 ms. T_2 in free water is also longer than that in bound water resulting in an increase in T_2 in lesions within tissue.

There has been some debate as to the reason behind the difference in relaxation times in the grey and white matter of the brain. Protons in lipids have a lower T_1 value, and the higher lipid content and lower water content of white versus grey matter was originally thought to be the explanation of the shorter T_1 in white matter compared with grey matter. However the form of the lipid will considerably influence the T_1 value. Lipids in bone marrow and scalp exist in the form of fatty acid triglycerides resulting in the relatively short T_1 of these tissues. However lipids in grey and white matter are mainly in the form of phospholipids which are highly immobilised resulting in a very short T_2 relaxation time.

A great deal of work has been carried out into the biological basis of T_1 and T_2 relaxation times both *in vivo* and *in vitro* at a variety of magnetic field strengths. A list of some typical T_1 values obtained *in vivo* is given in Table 2.2 and an extensive review of the subject has been published by Mathur-De Vré (1984).

Table 2.2 Normal human T_1 values (ms) measured *in vivo* at different magnetic field strengths

	Magnetic field strength (T)			
	0.04	0.08	0.15	1.5
Liver	140–170[1]	172–208	210–270[3]	
Spleen	250–290[1]	371–439	440–580[3]	
Grey matter	250–275[1]	392–438	340–610[4]	871 ± 73[5]
White matter	225–250[1]	265–292	220–350[4]	515 ± 27[5]
Cerebrospinal fluid	350–1000[2]		900–2000[4]	1900 ± 353[5]
Fat	120–140[1]	131–147		

[1] Hutchison and Smith (1983)
[2] Smith (1982)
[3] Straughan, Spencer and Bydder (1983)
[4] Bydder *et al.* (1982)
[5] Wehrli *et al.* (1984)

3

Pulse sequences

Introduction

We have seen in the previous chapter that the NMR signal has four separate components: the amplitude or size of the signal, the frequency, the phase and the duration of the resonance. If a single NMR signal is obtained from hydrogen nuclei within a sample then the amplitude of the signal is proportional to the proton density; no information about the T_1 or T_2 can be obtained from a single signal. However, if a sequence of RF pulses is used then the amplitude of the NMR signal can be changed so that it contains not only proton density information, but also information concerning the T_1 or T_2 of the sample. The timing and the sophistication of the pulse sequence results in different amounts of proton density, T_1 or T_2 information being contained in the amplitude of the NMR signal.

The amplitude of the NMR signal is eventually translated to an intensity value on an image. Thus the larger the amplitude of the NMR signal the brighter that particular part of a clinical image appears. It is the difference in amplitude of NMR signals from different parts of a section through the body which results in varying levels of brightness in the image and hence contrast. The signal amplitude is often therefore referred to as intensity, recognising that this is how it is finally displayed.

Saturation recovery

The simplest pulse sequence is called saturation recovery (also called partial saturation or repeated FID). Here 90° RF pulses are repeatedly applied to the sample and the NMR signal is measured after each RF pulse. The repetition time or time between pulses is referred to as *TR* (Fig. 3.1). If *TR* is relatively long, perhaps three or four times the T_1 of the sample, then all the nuclei have sufficient time to return to equilibrium before the next RF pulse. The amplitude of the NMR signal after each pulse therefore contains only proton density information. If, however, the pulse repetition time *TR* is much shorter, for example approximately equal to the T_1 of the sample, then the nuclei do not have sufficient time to return to their equilibrium position before the next RF pulse. The

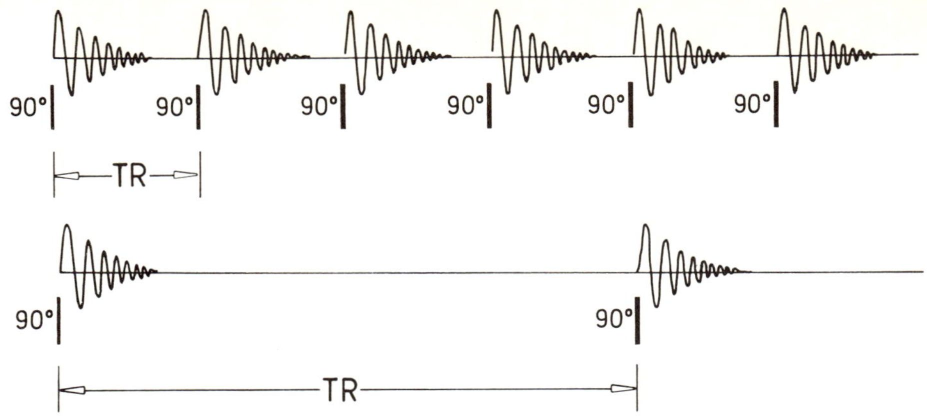

Fig. 3.1 Saturation recovery pulse sequences with a short repetition time *(TR)* and a long repetition time *(TR)*

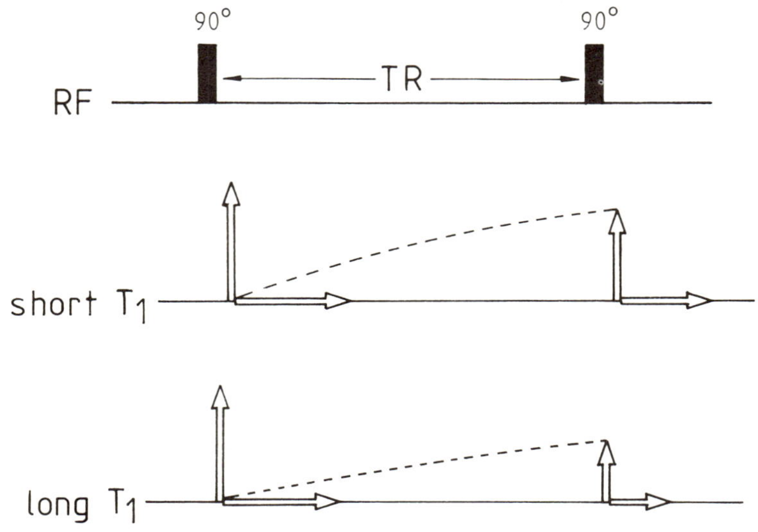

Fig. 3.2 Following a 90° pulse the component of magnetisation in the horizontal plane is the same magnitude as the component in the vertical direction prior to the application of the pulse. If following a 90° pulse a second 90° pulse is applied after a time *TR*, the vertical component of magnetisation may not have returned to its original size; the subsequent horizontal component will be correspondingly reduced, resulting in a smaller NMR signal. The effect of a short or long T_1 for a given *TR* is illustrated, the short T_1 sample resulting in a larger NMR signal being produced than the long T_1 sample

amplitude of the NMR signal is a function of the vertical component of magnetisation M_z prior to the application of the RF pulse. Thus if the nuclei in a sample are not given sufficient time to return to equilibrium their vertical component of magnetisation is reduced and hence the NMR signal is smaller. For any given value *TR* the amplitude of the NMR signals is influenced by the extent by which the nuclei have failed to return to equilibrium as illustrated in Fig. 3.2. Thus the amplitude of the NMR signal will contain information about the T_1 of the sample as well as the proton density, provided TR is short compared with T_1.

The amplitude of the NMR signal in the saturation recovery pulse sequence will be a function of proton density, TR and T_1. TR is the only variable in this sequence and it can be altered so that more or less T_1 information is contained in the signal. The faster the repetition time, that is the shorter the TR, the smaller the NMR signal becomes and the more T_1 information it contains. However, if the pulse repetition time is reduced too much the signal becomes so small that the quality of the final image becomes severely degraded.

Inversion recovery

The second pulse sequence we shall discuss produces NMR signals which potentially contain more T_1 information than saturation recovery. An example of the inversion recovery pulse sequence is illustrated in Fig. 3.3 and it can be seen that unlike the saturation recovery sequence, in this sequence two different RF pulses are applied before the NMR signal is produced, the pair of pulses being repeated every TR.

The principle of inversion recovery is very similar to that of saturation recovery. In both sequences the nuclei are not allowed sufficient time to return to equilibrium before the 90° pulse is applied. The difference is that in inversion recovery the nuclei are initially tipped through 180° rather than 90° as is used in the saturation recovery sequence. After the 180° pulse the magnetic moment M_z is large and negative rather than zero as it would be after a 90° pulse (Fig. 3.4). After the 180° pulse there is then a delay during which the nuclei will return to equilibrium, the value of M_z initially getting smaller, passing through the zero position then gradually increasing. The application of a 90° pulse during this return to equilibrium pro-

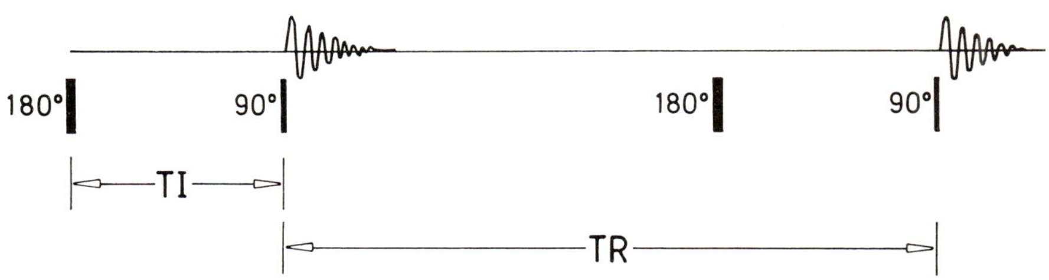

Fig. 3.3 Inversion recovery pulse sequence with a delay TI between the inverting 180° pulse and the subsequent 90° pulse. The repetition time of these pairs of pulses is TR

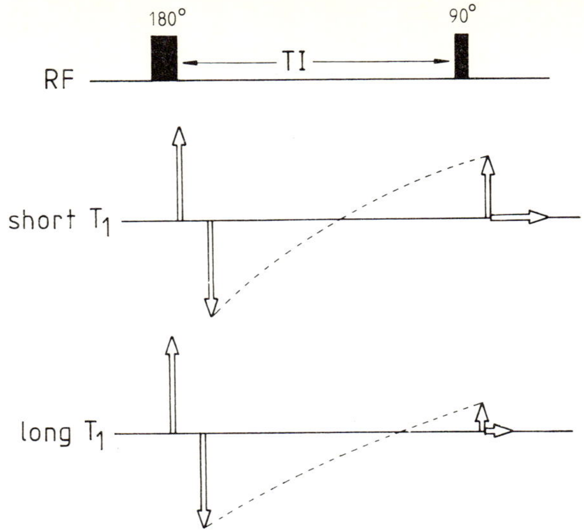

Fig. 3.4 Following a 180° pulse the nuclei are inverted. The vertical component of magnetisation then gets smaller, the variation in its magnitude with time being represented by the dotted lines. A short T_1 sample returns to equilibrium faster than a long T_1 sample, and so when the 90° pulse is applied the magnitude of the signal obtained is larger in the former than the latter. If *TI* had been half the value illustrated then the size of the signal from the sample with the short T_1 would be approximately zero, whereas the size of the original with the long T_1 would be larger though negative, producing a larger NMR signal

duces an NMR signal whose amplitude contains T_1 information, as it did in the case of the saturation recovery sequence, though more so. The time delay between the 180° and the 90° pulses determines the amount of T_1 information contained in the amplitude of the NMR signal, just as the time between successive 90° pulses did in the saturation recovery sequence. The time between the 180° and the 90° pulse is often referred to as tau (τ) or time from inversion (*TI*).

The amplitude of the NMR signal will be a function of the proton density, T_1, *TR* and *TI*. Though both of the last two variables influence the T_1 contribution in the final signal it is generally only the variable *TI* which is changed to influence the T_1 contribution. T_1 contrast in a clinical image is demonstrated much better with the inversion recovery sequence than with the saturation recovery sequence.

Spin echo

The spin echo pulse sequence produces an NMR signal in which both T_1 and T_2 contribute to the signal intensity. Although it contains information about both T_1 and T_2 it is principally to obtain

T_2 information that it is used in clinical investigations. The underlying physical principles of the spin echo pulse sequence are quite different from the previous two sequences that have been discussed and of the three pulse sequences it is perhaps the most difficult to understand.

We have seen in the previous chapter that the decay of the NMR signal is due to the loss of phase coherence in the precessing nuclei which in turn is caused by the minute variations in the magnetic field within the sample. Now there are two sources of this variation in the magnetic field: the precessing nuclei by themselves produce minor variations which are essentially random and there are also constant variations in the external magnetic field applied to the sample. Combinations of both these effects produce the T_2^* exponential decay of the NMR signal which is obtained in practice. It is sometimes convenient to refer to the exponential decay constants in terms of relaxation rates, the relaxation rate being simply the inverse of the relaxation time. The relaxation rates concerned with the loss of phase coherence are related as follows:

$$\frac{1}{T_2^*} = \frac{1}{T_2} + \frac{1}{T_2^{\text{magnet}}}$$

where T_2^{magnet} is the contribution to the loss of phase coherence caused by the inhomogeneities in the external magnetic field.

The spin echo pulse sequence utilises the fact that the component T_2^{magnet} is constant and therefore reversible. Following the application of a 90° pulse the nuclei initially precess in phase and then gradually lose phase coherence. If, however, after a short time interval a 180° pulse is applied the nuclei will be inverted about the x axis (using the coordinate convention that we have adopted) so that the positions of the faster and slower precessing nuclei are reversed. This is illustrated in Fig. 3.5. The effect of the inhomogeneities of the magnetic field on the loss of phase coherence of the nuclei is now reversed and so they gradually precess back into phase producing a large net magnetic moment and consequently an NMR signal. This signal occurs at the same time after the 180° pulse as the 180° was after the intitial 90° pulse. Because of the delay in the appearance of the signal it is referred to as an echo. The amplitude of the echo will be smaller than the original FID, which occurred immediately after the first 90° pulse, due to the irreversible loss of phase coherence caused by T_2. This process of rephasing the nuclei using 180° pulses can be repeated a number of times, the envelope described by all the echo signals being the true T_2 relaxation curve (Fig. 3.6).

The typical spin echo pulse sequence used for clinical imaging contains usually one or sometimes two 180° pulses as illustrated in Fig. 3.7. The time between the 90°, 180° pulse combination is *TR*

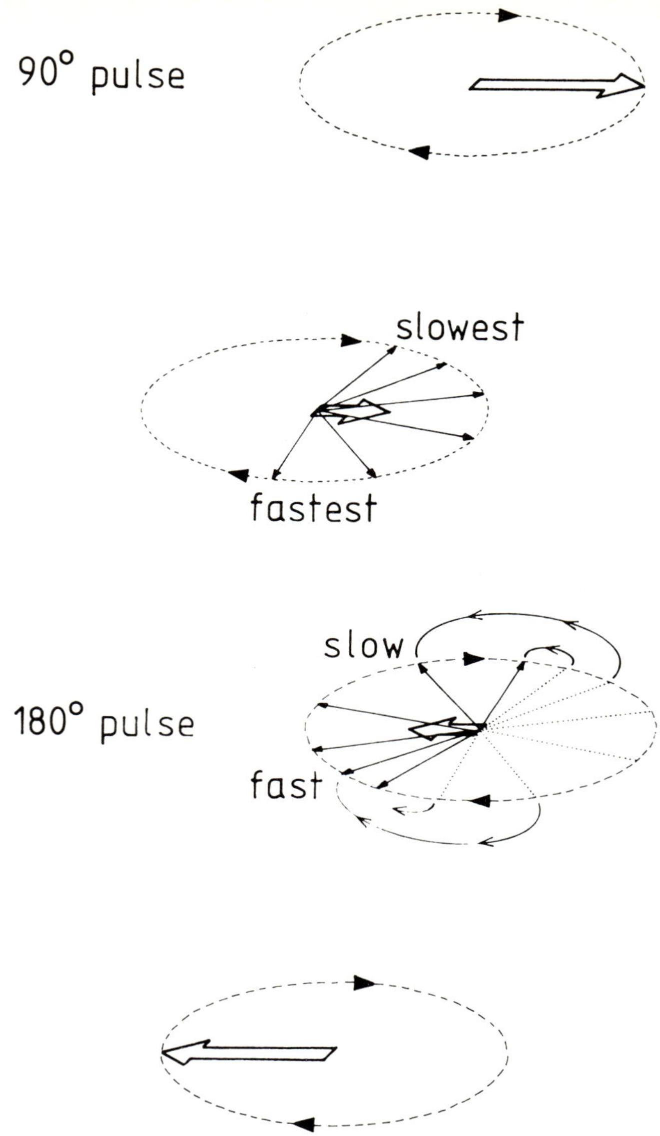

Fig. 3.5 Six nuclei in a sample initially precess in phase following a 90° pulse and so have a large net magnetic moment. After a time the net magnetic moment is reduced due to the gradual loss of phase coherence due to inhomogeneities in the magnetic field and to a small extent to spin–spin interactions. The application of a 180° pulse flips them about the x axis resulting in the relative positions of the slow and fast precessing nuclei becoming reversed. This results in the nuclei gradually coming into phase again increasing the horizontal component of magnetisation and producing an echo signal. The horizontal component of magnetisation is slightly smaller than the original horizontal component due to a loss of phase coherence from T_2

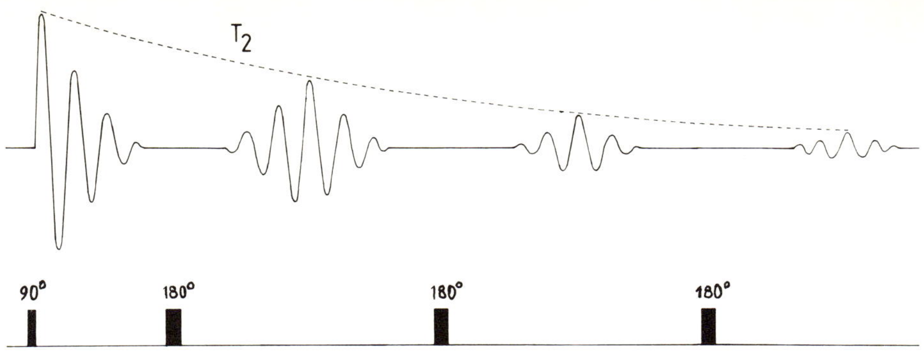

Fig. 3.6 Multiple spin echo pulse sequence. The NMR echoes occur at *TE*, 2 × *TE* and 3 × *TE* and the 180° pulses are applied at times *TE*/2, 3/2 × *TE*, 5/2 × *TE*. The envelope of the maximum values of the echoes is the T_2 relaxation curve

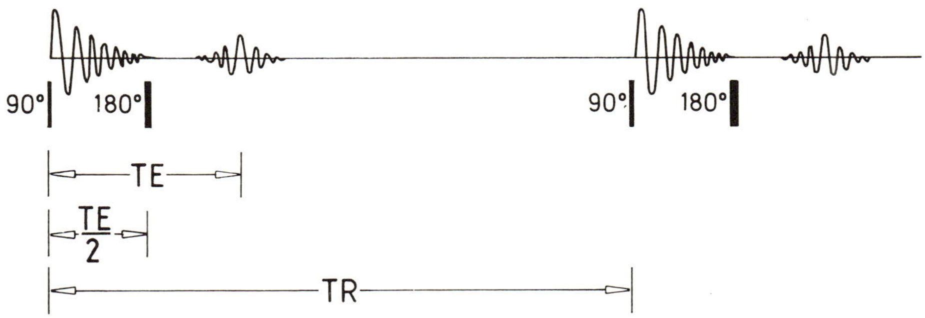

Fig. 3.7 Spin echo pulse sequence with the time to echo *(TE)* and the repetition time *(TR)*. The time between the 90° and the rephasing 180° pulse is *TE*/2

as in previous pulse sequences and as in the saturation recovery pulse sequence, the value of *TR* will determine the T_1 contribution in the echo signal. The time between the 90° and the echo signal is designated as *TE* and the larger this value the greater the T_2 contribution in the echo.

The amplitude of the NMR signal is therefore influenced by the variables proton density, T_1, T_2, *TR* and *TE*. The length of the delay *TE* is slightly less than an order of magnitude smaller than the delay *TI* in the inversion recovery pulse sequence. More details of how the timing of the various pulse sequences can influence the NMR signal will be discussed in detail later in this chapter (p.29).

T_1 and T_2 determination

The process of rephasing the nuclei using 180° pulse as described previously in the spin echo pulse sequence can be repeated a number

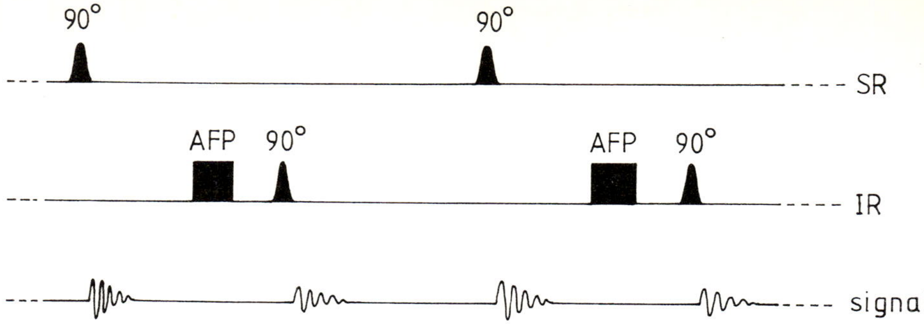

Fig. 3.8 Interleaved saturation recovery *(SR)* and inversion recovery *(IR)* pulse sequence used to produce two images from which a T_1 image can be calculated. Adiabatic fast passage *(AFP)* is a type of 180° pulse which inverts the nuclei very efficiently (see Chapter 5)

of times. The envelope so described by all the echo signals is the T_2 relaxation curve. This pulse sequence, which is illustrated in Fig. 3.6, is known as the Carr–Purcell sequence or, in its more recently modified form, as the Carr–Purcell–Meiboom–Gill (CPMG) sequence. The use of many echoes to determine the T_2 relaxation curve is necessary because it is likely that T_2 in biological samples may be multiexponential.

We have seen how a saturation recovery sequence with a sufficiently long *TR* can produce an NMR signal which contains only proton density information. When this pulse sequence is used in conjunction with an inversion recovery sequence, which contains both proton density and T_1 information, the T_1 value of a particular sample can be extracted. Figure 3.8 illustrates an interleaved saturation recovery and inversion recovery sequence which is used to produce two images from which a T_1 image can be calculated using the following equation (Edelstein *et al.*, 1980).

$$T_1 = TI / \ln \left[\frac{2I_{SR}}{I_{SR} - I_{IR}} \right]$$

where

I_{SR} = signal amplitude in saturation recovery image
I_{IR} = signal amplitude in inversion recovery image

It is also possible to calculate T_1 from repeated saturation recovery sequences, each with different *TR* or from repeated inversion recovery sequences each with a different *TI*. These methods are sometimes used although they can be fairly time-consuming.

Effect of sequence timing on NMR signal size

In MRI the intensity of a part of an image will be a function of the amplitude of the NMR signal from that region. It is important therefore to understand how the timing values *TR*, *TE* and *TI* can affect the relative contributions of proton density, T_1 or T_2 in the NMR signal and hence alter the appearance and contrast of the final image. Some MRI systems use a fixed pulse sequence and obtain a T_1 image. Most systems, however, give the operator the option of choosing the timing values *TR*, *TE* and *TI*, depending on the pulse sequence used, so that the maximum contrast between the particular tissues of interest is obtained. This presupposes that the T_1 and T_2 values of the tissues are known to some extent so that the timing can be chosen to produce the maximum contrast.

The fact that the T_1 of a tissue is not constant but increases as the strength of the magnet used for MRI increases complicates the problem of pulse sequence timing still further. The optimum pulse sequence timing for a certain pathological condition will vary depending on the field strength of the main magnet of the MRI system. Values of *TR* vary from 200 ms to 3000 ms, with the majority of scans being performed with values between 1000 ms and 2000 ms. Values of *TI* vary from 200 ms to 1200 ms and values of *TE* vary from 20 ms to 100 ms. The order of magnitude difference between values *TI* and *TE* makes it obvious as to which timing interval a number refers. It is usual to quote the sequence timing for any clinical image simply as two or three numbers, the timing always being quoted in milliseconds (ms) and in a specific order. Examples and explanations of this convention are given below:

1500,400	Inversion recovery sequence: $TR = 1500$ ms, $TI = 400$ ms
1600,56	Spin echo sequence: $TR = 1600$ ms, $TE = 56$ ms
2000,30,500	Inversion recovery sequence with a further 180° pulse soon after the 90° pulse to produce an echo: $TR = 2000$ ms, $TE = 30$ ms, $TI = 500$ ms

TR is always listed first and when only two numbers are present it is possible by the size of the second number to infer whether it is an inversion recovery sequence or a spin echo sequence. In an inversion recovery sequence with a spin echo after the 90° pulse there will be three numbers which define the pulse sequence. These are often listed in the order *TR*, *TE*, then *TI*.

The amplitude of the NMR signal and hence the intensity of a particular point in an image can be obtained from the following equations for the three fundamental pulse sequences:

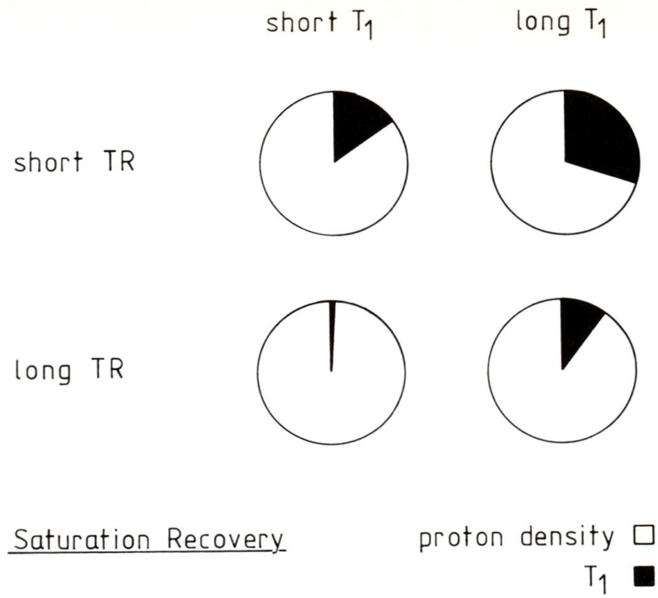

Fig. 3.9 The relative contributions to the NMR signal intensity using a saturation recovery pulse sequence

$$\text{Saturation recovery} \quad I_{SR} = k\rho \left[1 - e^{-\frac{TR}{T_1}}\right]$$

$$\text{Inversion recovery} \quad I_{IR} = k\rho \left[1 - 2e^{-\frac{TI}{T_1}} + e^{-\frac{TR}{T_1}}\right]$$

$$\text{Spin echo} \quad I_{SE} = k\rho \left[1 - e^{-\frac{TR}{T_1}}\right] e^{-\frac{TE}{T_2}}$$

where

I	= signal amplitude or intensity of point on the image
ρ	= proton density
TR	= repetition time, between 90° pulses
TI	= time from inversion, between 180° and 90° pulses
TE	= time to echo
T_1	= T_1 value of sample or point in the image
T_2	= T_2 value of sample or point in the image

The amplitude of the NMR signal and hence the intensity of any region of an image will contain different amounts of proton density, T_1 and T_2 information depending not only on their respective values but also on the timing of the pulse sequence used. The relative contributions of proton density, T_1 and T_2 can be represented using a 'pie' diagram, in which the respective sizes of the segments represent the relative contributions to the intensity of the image. These can be calculated exactly using the equations above for any given situation. However, in order to understand the differences between

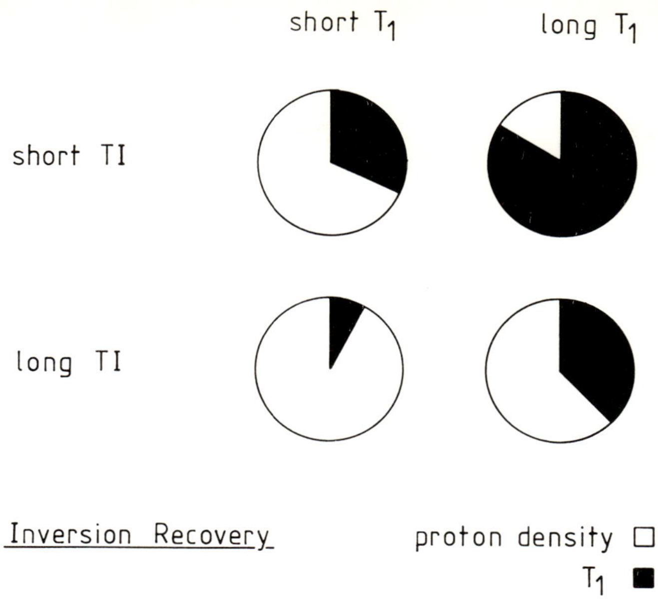

Fig. 3.10 Relative contributions to the NMR signal intensity from an inversion recovery pulse sequence

the pulse sequences, we will simply consider the example of short and long T_1 and T_2 and short and long *TR*, *TE*, and *TI*.

The effect of short and long *TR* on a saturation recovery sequence is illustrated in Fig. 3.9. As can be seen, when a long *TR* is used on a region of the body with a short T_1 then the image obtained will be essentially a proton density image, the intensity of the signal containing only a very small amount of T_1 information. In the same section the amount of T_1 information in the image will gradually increase as *TR* is reduced. A long *TR* is often chosen to obtain a proton density image, but as can be seen in Fig. 3.9 the T_1 information will be present using a long *TR* if the T_1 itself is long. This explains why proton density images of the brain using a long *TR* show cerebrospinal fluid (CFS) to have relatively low proton density; this is due to the relatively long T_1 of the CSF compared with the rest of the brain and consequent reduction in the signal intensity.

Figure 3.10 illustrates the effect of short and long *TI* in the inversion recovery sequence, assuming that a long *TR* has been used. As can be seen the relationship between short and long T_1 and the pulse timing *TI* is similar to the relationship in Fig. 3.9 for saturation recovery. However, the T_1 contribution to the signal is much greater using inversion recovery, and as a consequence it is the sequence of choice when wishing to highlight contrast between tissues of different T_1 values. The term 'contrast' simply refers to the difference between two NMR signal values which is presented as the difference

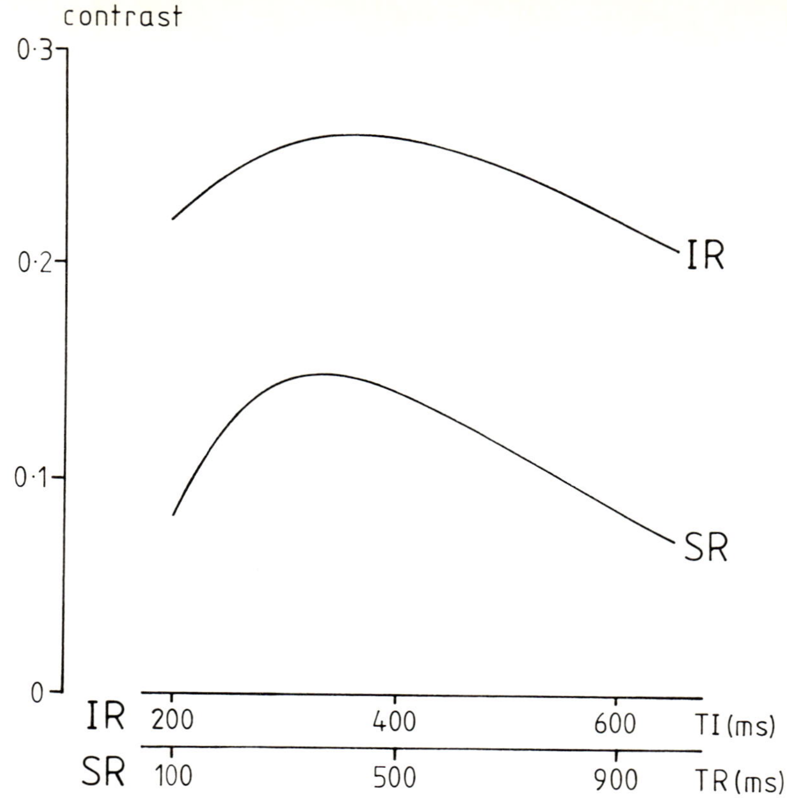

Fig. 3.11 The difference in NMR signal intensities (that is, contrast) between tissues with different T_1 values using inversion recovery *(IR)* or saturation recovery *(SR)* pulse sequences. The two curves show the contrast between tissues with a T_1 at 300 ms and 450 ms, approximately the values for white and grey matter respectively at a field strength of 0.15 T. In the inversion recovery sequence a *TR* of 1400 ms is used. The higher contrast between the two tissues using the inversion recovery sequence is clearly demonstrated

in intensity of an image on a screen, or as the difference in film density if the image has been transferred to transparent film. The superiority of inversion recovery over saturation recovery is highlighted in Fig. 3.11 in which the contrast between two different tissues of different T_1 values (grey and white matter in the brain) is illustrated for different values of *TR* and *TI* in the saturation recovery and inversion recovery sequence respectively.

So far the two pulse sequences considered contain only proton density and T_1 information in the signal intensity. The spin echo pulse sequence (Fig. 3.12) is more complex because it contains T_2 information in addition to proton density and T_1 information, and both *TR* and *TE* are varied to influence the relative contribution. A long *TR* is used to reduce the amount of T_1 information in the

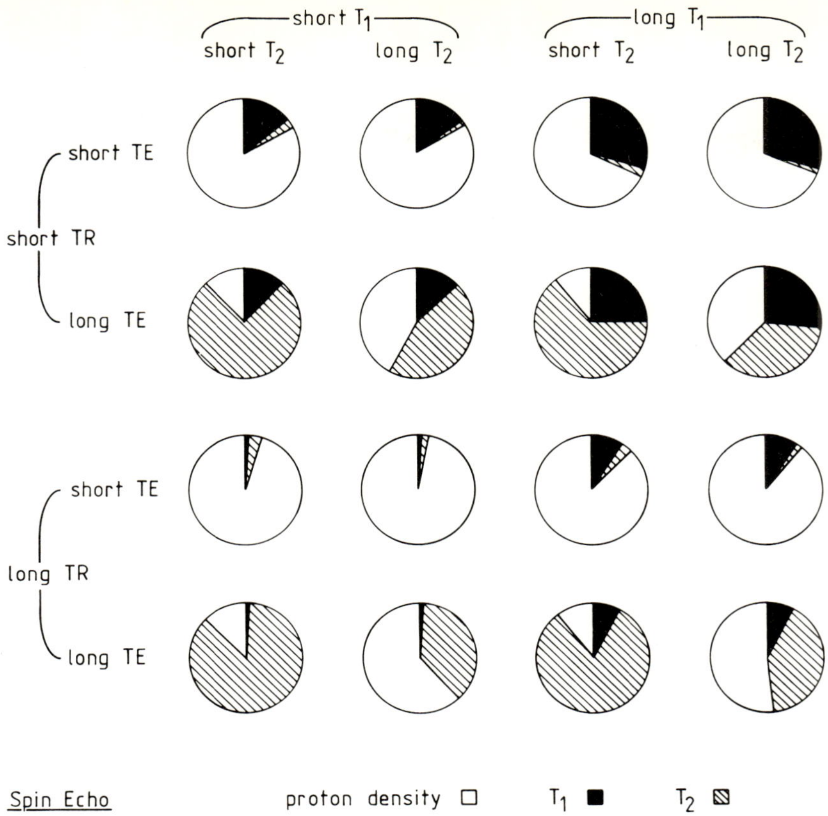

Fig. 3.12 Relative NMR signal intensities using a spin echo pulse sequence

image as much as possible in conjunction with a short *TE* to obtain essentially a proton density image or alternatively a long *TE* to obtain a heavily weighted T_2 image. A reduction of *TR* will increase the amount of T_1 information in the intensity whereas a reduction in *TE* will reduce the amount of T_2 information.

A fourth pulse sequence is an inversion recovery with a spin echo. The effect of varying *TR*, *TE* and *TI* is analogous to the previously described spin echo example except that *TI* is varied instead of *TR* to obtain T_1 information. The increase in T_1 information is the same as the increase between a simple saturation recovery sequence and a simple inversion recovery sequence (compare Figs. 3.9 and 3.10).

The effect of different pulse sequences and their timing on the appearance of an image is dramatically illustrated in Fig. 3.13. The variation in contrast between normal and abnormal tissue in the liver can be seen, in particular the ability of the lesion to 'disappear' with a particular sequence.

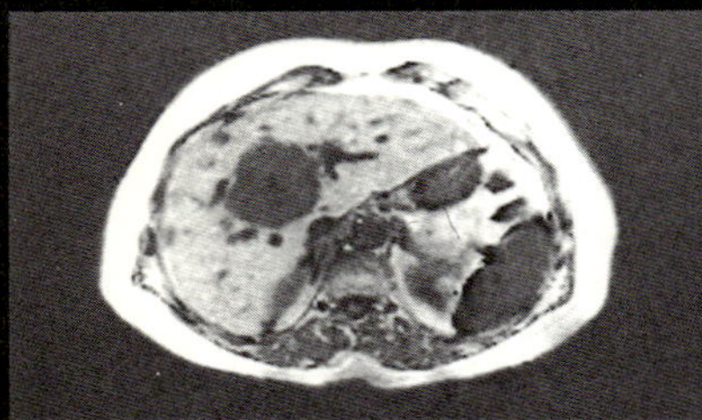

(a)

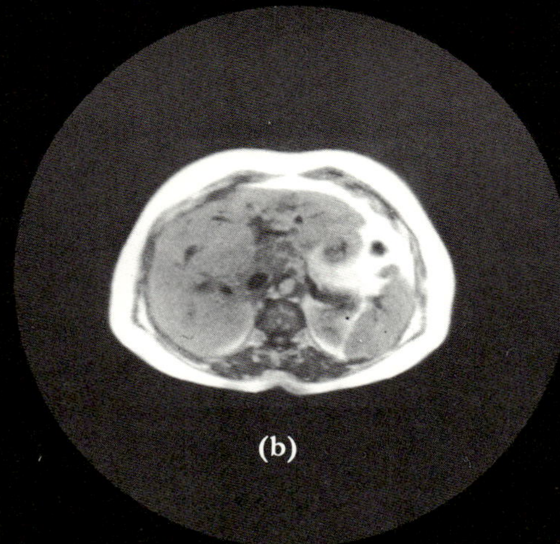

(b)

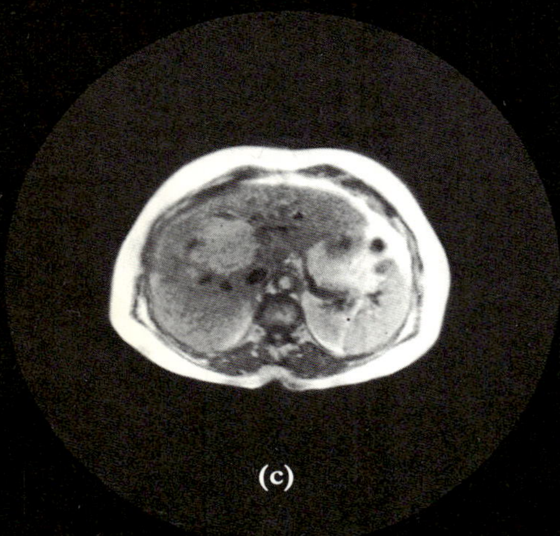

(c)

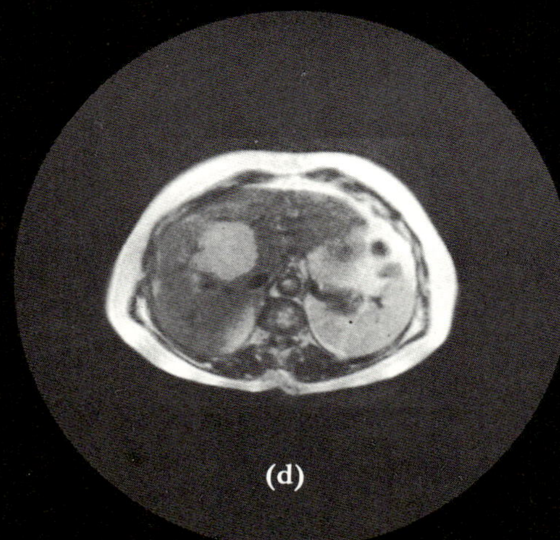

(d)

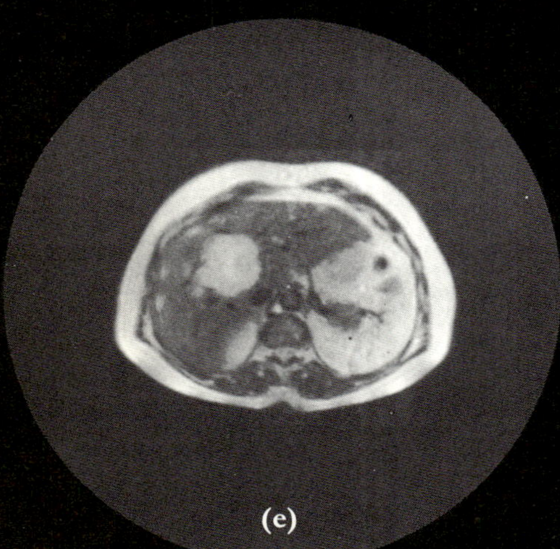

(e)

Fig. 3.13 Effect of pulse sequence and timing on the contrast between a lesion in the liver and normal tissue. *(a)* Inversion recovery: *TR* = 1400, *TI* = 400. The other images are spin echo: *(b) TR* = 540, *TE* = 20; *(c) TR* = 1040, *TE* = 20; *(d) TR* = 1080, *TE* = 40; and *(e) TR* = 2080, *TE* = 40 (courtesy of Hammersmith Hospital, London)

4

Image production

Introduction

To obtain images of tomographic sections through large samples such as the human body using NMR, two different approaches can be adopted. The first is when resonance is produced in a small volume of the sample, for example a cube of 1 cm^3, so that any signal detected is known to come from that small region of known position. This selected region can then be moved in such a way that the NMR signals detected gradually build up a map of a tomographic section. The second and far more sensitive approach is when resonance is produced in a much larger volume and spatial information is stored within the NMR signal itself.

One fundamental aspect of different imaging techniques is the dimension of the sample from which an NMR signal is acquired which serves as a useful classification of different imaging techniques. Imagine a cube as illustrated in Fig. 4.1 which contains n voxels (a voxel is a volume element, the three-dimensional equivalent of a pixel) over each side such that its total volume is n^3. There are four imaging categories, the first being single point, sometimes called sequential point (Fig. 4.1(*a*)) where the NMR signal comes from 1 voxel. The second is the line technique (Fig. 4.1(*b*)) where the NMR signal comes from a line of n voxels. Early imaging techniques used single point or line methods but both of these are relatively inefficient as the NMR signal is produced from a relatively small number of nuclei. The third and most commonly used method of image production is the planar technique (Fig. 4.1(*c*)) where the NMR signal is obtained from a plane of n^2 voxels within the volume. The fourth method is the volume imaging technique (Fig. 4.1(*d*)) where the NMR signal comes from all n^3 voxels within the volume.

Magnetic gradients

Up till now we have only considered the production of an NMR signal in the presence of a strong, constant, uniform magnetic field H_0. However, fundamental to all techniques of MRI is the use of additional, much smaller, magnetic fields which can be switched on

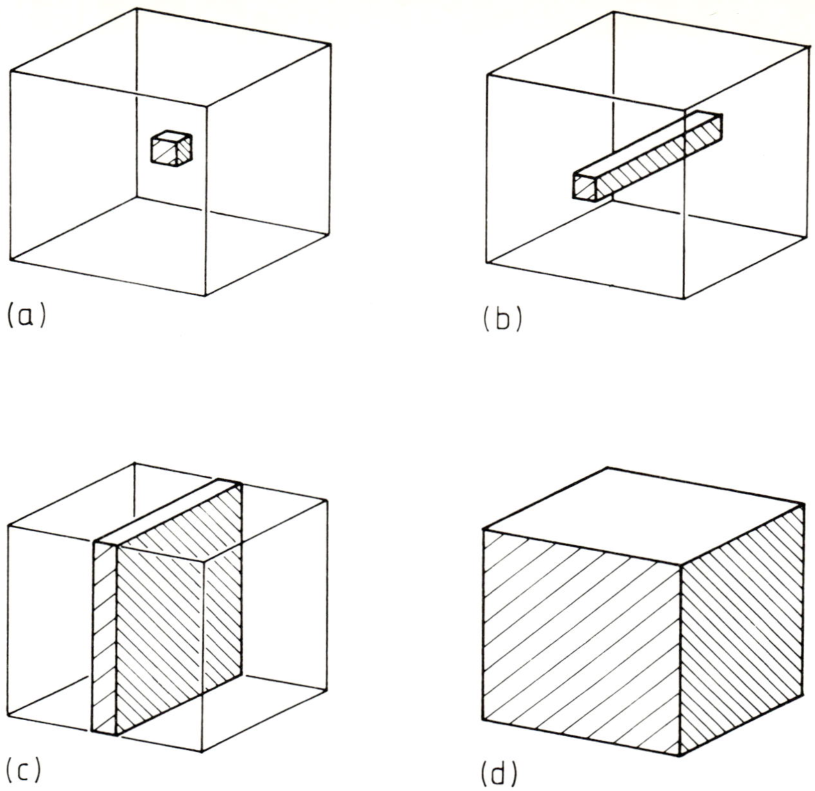

Fig. 4.1 Four imaging categories: *(a)* single point, *(b)* line, *(c)* planar and *(d)* volume

and off fairly rapidly. These additional magnetic fields take the form of linear gradient fields in the x, y and z coordinate directions. These magnetic fields are designated by the terms G_x, G_y and G_z, and although their amplitudes vary linearly in the three coordinate directions, the direction of all three gradient fields is in the same direction as the main constant magnetic field. An example of a gradient field is illustrated in Fig. 4.2. It can be seen that the gradient field varies linearly from a negative value on the left to a positive value on the right, the thickness of the arrows representing the fact that the variation in the magnetic field along the gradient is about 100 times smaller than the main magnetic field value. As the gradient field value is fairly low it is possible to switch gradient fields on and off fairly quickly. It will be seen later that this is necessary for image production. The total magnetic field experienced by a patient will be the main magnetic field plus the gradient field, and as can be seen in Fig. 4.2 this will result in a total field with a small linear variation across the patient.

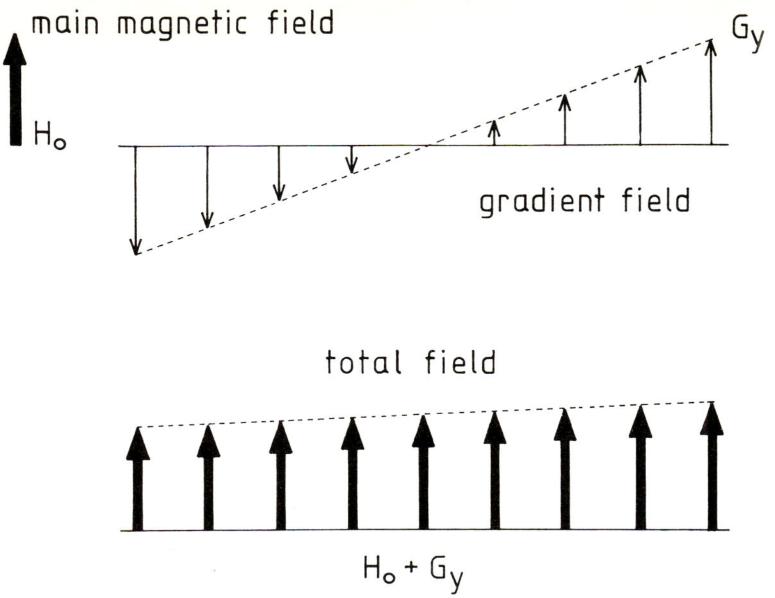

Fig. 4.2 Gradient field G_y superimposed on the main magnetic field H_0; the total field has a shallow linear variation in the y coordinate direction

Selective excitation

As its name suggests this is a technique by which resonance can be produced within a selected region of a larger sample. Imagine a sample such as the human body placed in a strong external magnetic field H_0 (Fig. 4.3). This external magnetic field is effectively constant along the length of the patient. A magnetic field gradient is now applied, much weaker than the external magnetic field, which is in the same direction but which varies along the length of the patient. In Fig. 4.3 it can be seen that the magnetic gradient is such that this second magnetic field is lower at the patient's head and higher at the patient's feet. The total magnetic field experienced by the body is the sum of the magnetic gradient field plus the external magnetic field, so the total magnetic field varies along the length of the patient from H_1 at the head increasing to H_5 at the feet. We know that the frequency of resonance is directly related to the magnetic field and so the Larmor resonant frequency of the nuclei will vary in a linear fashion in the same way, being lower at the head ω_1 and higher at the feet ω_5. A situation now exists where different frequencies must be applied to produce resonance in different parts of the body. If we therefore apply RF with a frequency ω_3 only nuclei within a transverse section at that corresponding part of the body will resonate. If we were to apply a frequency ω_4 we would obtain

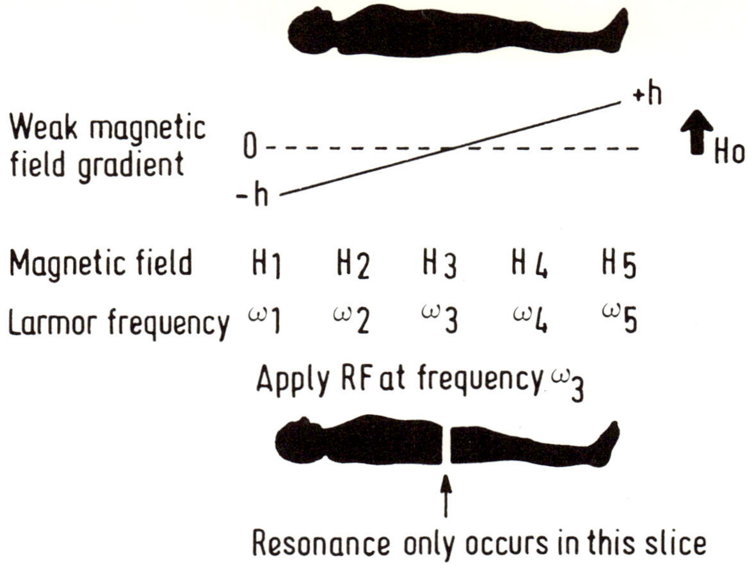

Fig. 4.3 Principal of selective excitation. The total magnetic field linearly increases from H_1 at the head to H_5 at the feet with a corresponding linear variation in the Larmor frequency of resonance. The application of RF at frequency ω_3 results in resonance occurring in a transverse tomographic section in the body with Larmor frequency ω_3

a transverse slice through the knees, likewise ω_1 would give a transverse slice through the head.

It would of course be possible to apply simultaneously a magnetic gradient *across* the patient in addition to the magnetic gradient *along* the patient so that instead of resonance being induced in a plane, it would be produced in a line. If, in addition, a third magnetic gradient were also applied in the remaining coordinate direction, resonance could be produced at just a single point. In almost all MRI systems the technique of selective excitation is used to select the plane to be imaged and so a single magnetic gradient is used. A sagittal tomographic section can be selected by using a magnetic gradient across the patient, likewise a coronal section can be selected by using a gradient which varies from front to back.

In Fig. 4.3 it was seen how the application of a single RF frequency selected the transverse slice. It is not possible to transmit a single RF frequency, there always being a range of frequencies however small. This narrow range of frequencies is referred to as the bandwidth and it is this, combined with the steepness of the magnetic gradient, which determines the width of the section selected. If the magnetic gradient were increased then the RF bandwidth would also have to be increased to maintain a constant width of the section selected. It follows therefore that if the bandwidth remains constant then the thickness of the slice can be varied by increasing or decreasing the slope of the magnetic field gradient.

Frequency encoded spatial information

In the preceding chapter it was demonstrated how T_1 and T_2 information can be stored in the amplitude of the NMR signal by the use of appropriate pulse sequences. Up to this point the phase and the frequency of the NMR signal have not been used in MRI for any purpose. One of the fundamental developments of MRI was the use of these two components of the NMR signal to store spatial information. Using selective excitation, NMR signals are produced from a two-dimensional slice within the patient; the frequency of the signal is then used to store spatial information in one dimension and the phase of the NMR signal used to store spatial information in the other dimension.

Spatial information is stored in the NMR signal using another magnetic field gradient which is applied while the NMR signal is actually being received rather than while the resonance is being induced as in the case of selective excitation. The principle of frequency encoded spatial information also relies on the linear relationship between the frequency of resonance and the magnetic field. This means that although all the nuclei in a section precess at the same frequency immediately after selective excitation, if the overall magnetic field is varied in any way thereafter the frequencies of resonance of the nuclei within the slice will not remain the same but will vary according to the magnetic field.

The principle is best understood diagrammatically and is illustrated in Fig. 4.4. Resonance is induced in a transverse section by selective excitation using a magnetic gradient along the length of the patient. Immediately after this a magnetic gradient is applied perpendicular to the gradient used for selective excitation, as shown in Fig. 4.4. In the example the transverse section contains two circles of resonating nuclei. If the magnetic field gradient is applied during the detection of the NMR signal it can be seen that the two samples experience separate magnetic fields and therefore resonate at quite separate frequencies. The NMR signal detected therefore contains not just one frequency, as would be the case if no gradient had been applied, but two. This is shown in the hypothetical NMR signal illustrated in Fig. 4.4, where the higher frequency ω_2 is seen superimposed on the lower frequency ω_1. The frequency information of any signal can be extracted using a mathematical technique called Fourier transform as illustrated in Fig. 4.5. If the NMR signal

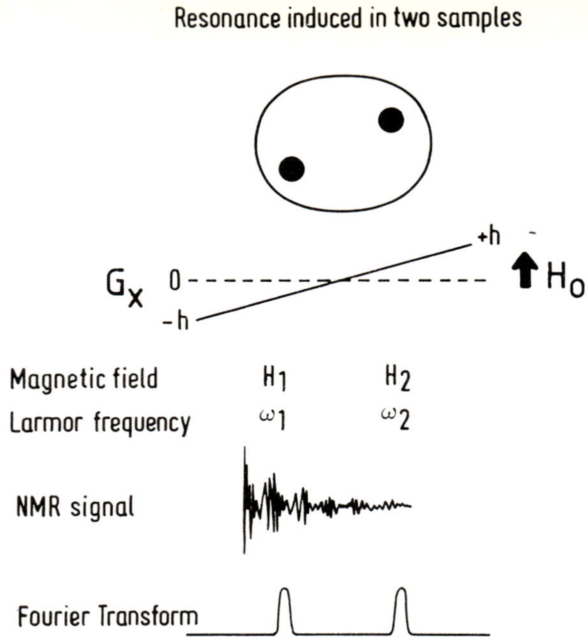

Fig. 4.4 Frequency encoded spatial information. The detection of the NMR signal in the presence of a linearly varying magnetic field will cause the two samples to resonate at different frequencies. The detected NMR signal then contains these two frequencies which can be extracted using the mathematical technique of Fourier transformation

in Fig. 4.4 is Fourier transformed the result is two peaks corresponding to the frequencies ω_1 and ω_2. With appropriate calibration the position of these peaks will correspond with the position of the two samples in the transverse slice. If the left-hand sample had been further to the left then its corresponding frequency would be lower, and so after Fourier transformation of the NMR signal the left-hand peak would be further to the left by an amount corresponding to the change in position of the sample. Using the magnetic gradient during the detection of the NMR signal the position across the transverse slice is therefore going to be uniquely related to a particular frequency, and so after Fourier transformation a projection of the section is obtained.

A third magnetic field gradient, perpendicular to the two gradients already discussed, applied at the same time as the frequency encoded gradient can produce a one-dimensional projection of the tomographic section from any angle. An image can therefore be constructed using conventional back projection techniques similar to those used in X-ray CT. The back projection method was one of the earlier techniques used for NMR image production and though it has largely been superseded it is still occasionally used in some

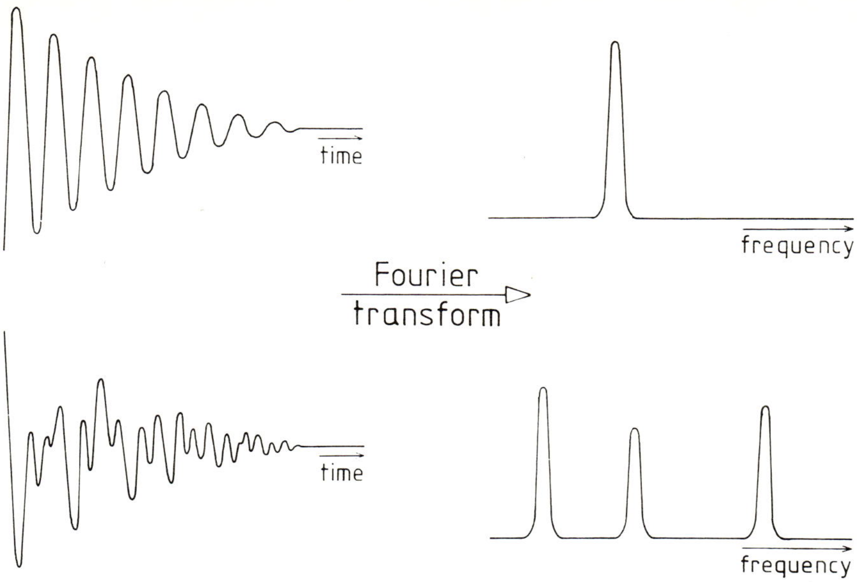

Fig. 4.5 An NMR signal is a varying amplitude in the time domain. We wish to convert such a signal to the frequency domain in which the relative proportion of different frequencies can be displayed. This can be done using a Fourier transform. The upper NMR signal consists of a single frequency, and so following Fourier transformation a single peak will be displayed. The lower signal is more complex and following Fourier transformation it can be seen that it contains three different proportions

MRI systems. The disadvantages of the back projection method of image reconstruction are its relative intolerance of patient movement and magnetic field inhomogeneity, although it may have some advantages in terms of spatial resolution.

Two-dimensional Fourier transform

The technique which has become standard for single slice image production is that of two-dimensional Fourier transform (2DFT), a particular form of which is also known as 'spin-warp' (Edelstein *et al.*, 1980). This method of image production uses the frequency to store spatial information in one dimension of a tomographic section and the phase of the NMR signal to store spatial information in the other dimension; 2DFT involving the phase encoding of spatial information is one of the more difficult concepts to grasp in the field of MRI.

The technique of phase encoded spatial information is always used in conjunction with frequency encoding in the other dimensions but at this stage we shall simply consider how spatial information can be stored in the phase of the signal. Remember that the convention of MRI is that the z coordinate direction is the direction of the main magnetic field H_0. So far in this chapter we have taken H_0 to be in the vertical direction and we will continue with this convention. Assume that a magnetic gradient G_y has been applied to resonate selectively a transverse tomographic section and subsequently the gradient G_x is switched on during the signal detection period to frequency encode the spatial information in the x direction. These two gradients G_y and G_x are applied at different times, during the so-called excitation and detection periods respectively, between which there is a time interval known as the evolution period. It is during this evolution period that the remaining gradient G_z is applied to encode the spatial information in the z direction in the phase of the NMR signal. During the application of the phase encoding gradient G_z, the nuclei within the section precess at different frequencies as described by the Larmor equation; the nuclei at the top of the section will precess faster than the nuclei at the bottom of the section. This results in a varying phase angle throughout the z direction of the section, and at any instant the phase angle at the top of the section will be larger than the phase angle at the bottom, with a linear variation through the section. When the gradient G_z is switched off the variation in phase in the z direction will be maintained even though all the nuclei will have reverted to the same frequency of precession.

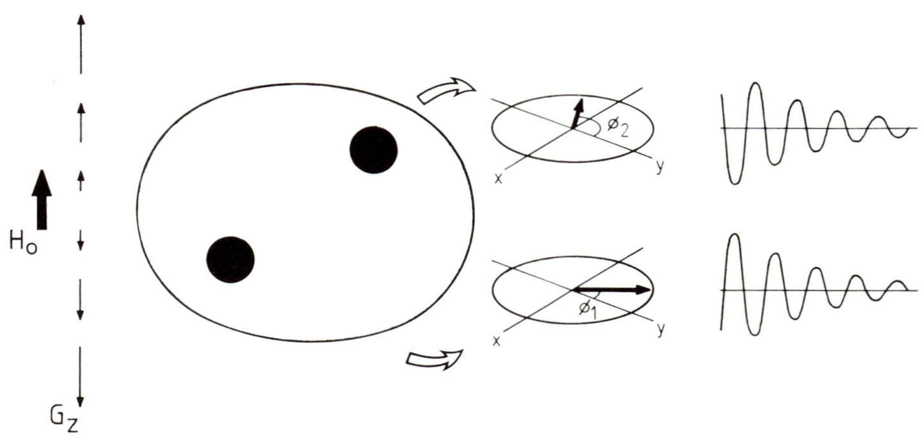

Fig. 4.6 Phase encoded spatial information. The application of a gradient G_z during the time period between excitation and detection of the signal will cause the two samples in the tomographic section to precess at different frequencies corresponding to the total magnetic field which is larger towards the top of the section and smaller towards the bottom of the section. When the gradient is switched off the two samples precess at the same frequency but with different phase angles, ϕ_1 for the lower sample and ϕ_2 for the upper sample. The NMR signal obtained from the two samples separately therefore has a different phase, the phase being related to the position in the slice

This variation in phase angle is translated to the NMR signal as illustrated in Fig. 4.6.

It is not too difficult to perceive how the phase of the NMR signal can be used to store spatial information, but now consider how this information is extracted by the use of a Fourier transform in the second dimension. So far during NMR image production we have seen that a sequence of pulses is used to obtain T_1 or T_2 information and for each NMR signal the identical G_y for selective excitation and G_x for frequency encoding is used. However, to extract the phase information a different amplitude G_z gradient pulse is applied for each NMR signal. The amplitude or duration of the phase encoding gradient gradually changes during a scan. It does not matter whether the amplitude or duration changes, the effect is the same; the variation in phase angle due to position in the z direction will be different for each NMR signal. In Fig. 4.7(*a*) the successive NMR signals from the sample towards the bottom of the section are arranged in a column. The field from the G_z gradient value at this level is fairly small and though the slope of the gradient itself gradually increases for successive NMR signals the change in phase angle is fairly small. A plot of the amplitude of the NMR signals corresponding to a vertical line drawn through them will result in a low frequency variation. Similarly, in Fig. 4.7(*b*) the sample at the top of the section experiencing a larger effect of the phase encoding gradient is considered. As the slope of the gradient is increased for successive NMR signals there will be a much greater absolute variation in magnetic field, and consequently phase angle, between the different signals. The plot of the amplitudes of the NMR signals along a corresponding vertical line to Fig. 4.7(*a*) results in a variation of higher frequency. By considering the signals one on top of another and taking vertical sections through them, the variation in phase angle at different positions in the z direction through the section will correspond to variations in frequency. This frequency is linearly related to the spatial position in the z direction and consequently the latter can be extracted using a Fourier transform.

A typical RF and gradient sequence for 2DFT is illustrated in Fig. 4.8. A number of NMR signals, usually 64, 128 or 256, are detected and a different amplitude of G_z is used for each signal. Each digitised signal from each value of the G_z gradient will be stored one above the other to form a two-dimensional array (Fig. 4.9(*a*)). It can be seen that this array of raw NMR data is symmetrical in both the x and z directions. The final image is obtained from a two-dimensional Fourier transform of this data (Fig. 4.9(*b*)).

The time taken to acquire a single section will depend on three factors: (*a*) the timing of the pulse sequences used, in particular the value TR; (*b*) the number of different G_z phase encoding gradients

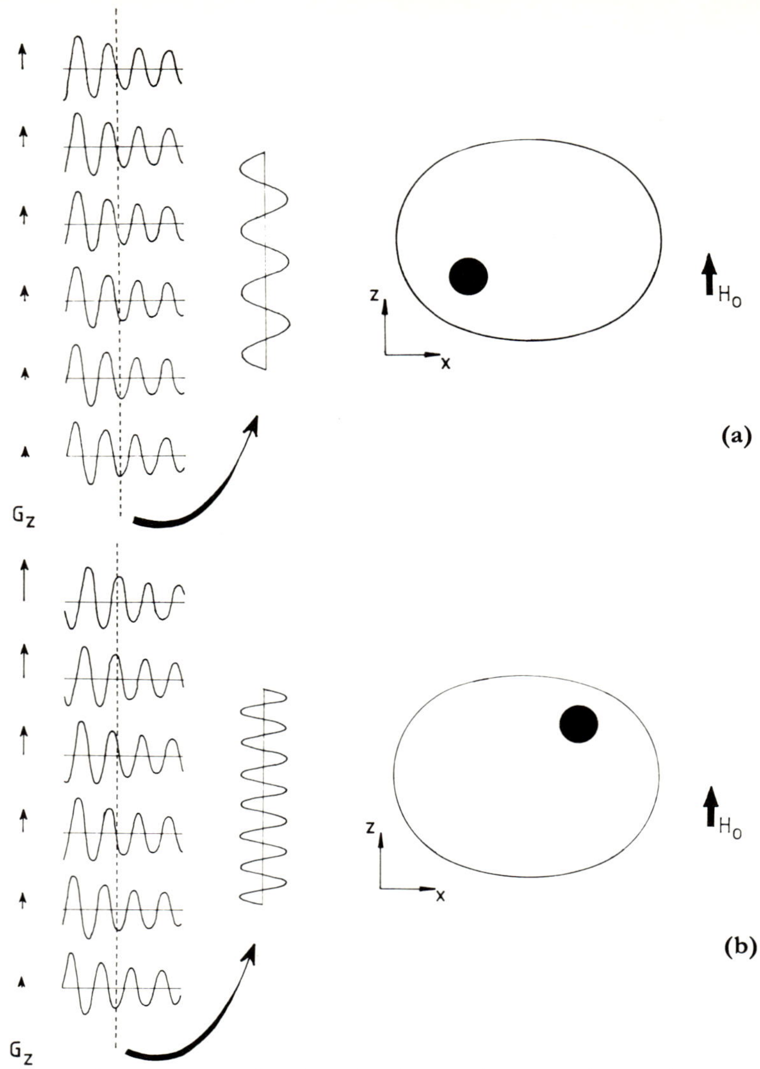

Fig. 4.7 During the production of an image a large number, perhaps 128, of different G_z phase encoding gradients are applied. Consider the magnetic field experienced by a sample at the bottom *(a)* and top *(b)* of the slice during six of these 128 different values of G_z. During these successive gradients the magnetic field at the top of the section will increase faster than the magnetic field at the bottom of the section resulting in the sample at the top of the section experiencing a greater phase change during this period than the sample at the bottom of this section. If the NMR signals detected from the two samples considered separately are placed one above the other the amplitude of the signals at a particular time is represented by the vertical dotted lines. Plotting the amplitude of the signals where they cross this dotted line results in an oscillating curve whose frequency is *(b)* larger where the phase change is larger, and *(a)* smaller where the phase change is smaller

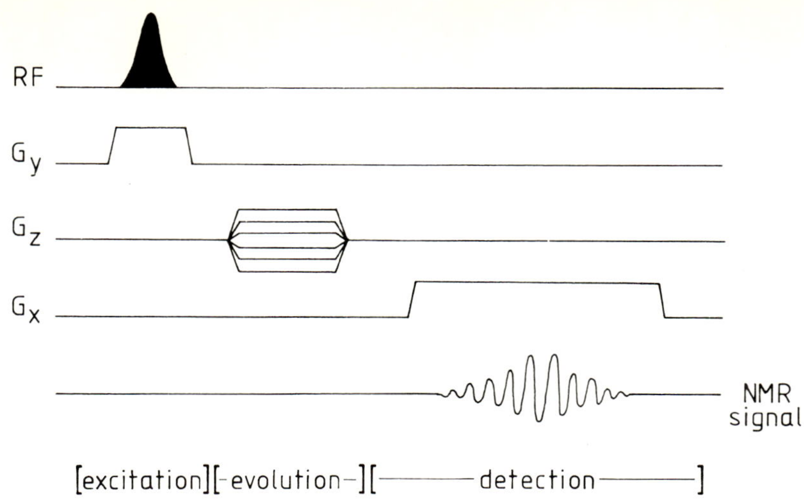

Fig. 4.8 RF and gradient pulse sequence for two-dimensional Fourier transform (2DFT)

used, whether 64, 128 or 256; and (*c*) the number of times the NMR signal is recorded for each gradient value, the average of several signals giving improved resolution. The shortest acquisition time is of the order of 10 s for a saturation recovery sequence with short *TR*, 64 different G_z gradients and no signal averaging (that is, a single signal for each gradient). An example of an image with a long acquisition time would be an inversion recovery sequence with $TR = 1400$, $TI = 400$, 256 G_z gradients and four signal averages. This would result in a high resolution image taking 30 min to acquire.

Simultaneous acquisition

So far the production of an image of a single tomographic section has been considered. For most clinical situations however, information is usually required from a volume within the patient; in X-ray CT this is done by performing a number of tomographic sections one after the other, moving the patient between each section. This of course can also be done using MRI but, because of the longer acquisition time per section, the time taken to obtain information from a volume within a patient can be longer than with X-ray CT. However, there are two more efficient methods of obtaining information from a volume within a patient using MRI; these are called (*a*) simultaneous slice acquisition or sometimes multiple slice acquisition, and (*b*) volume acquisition.

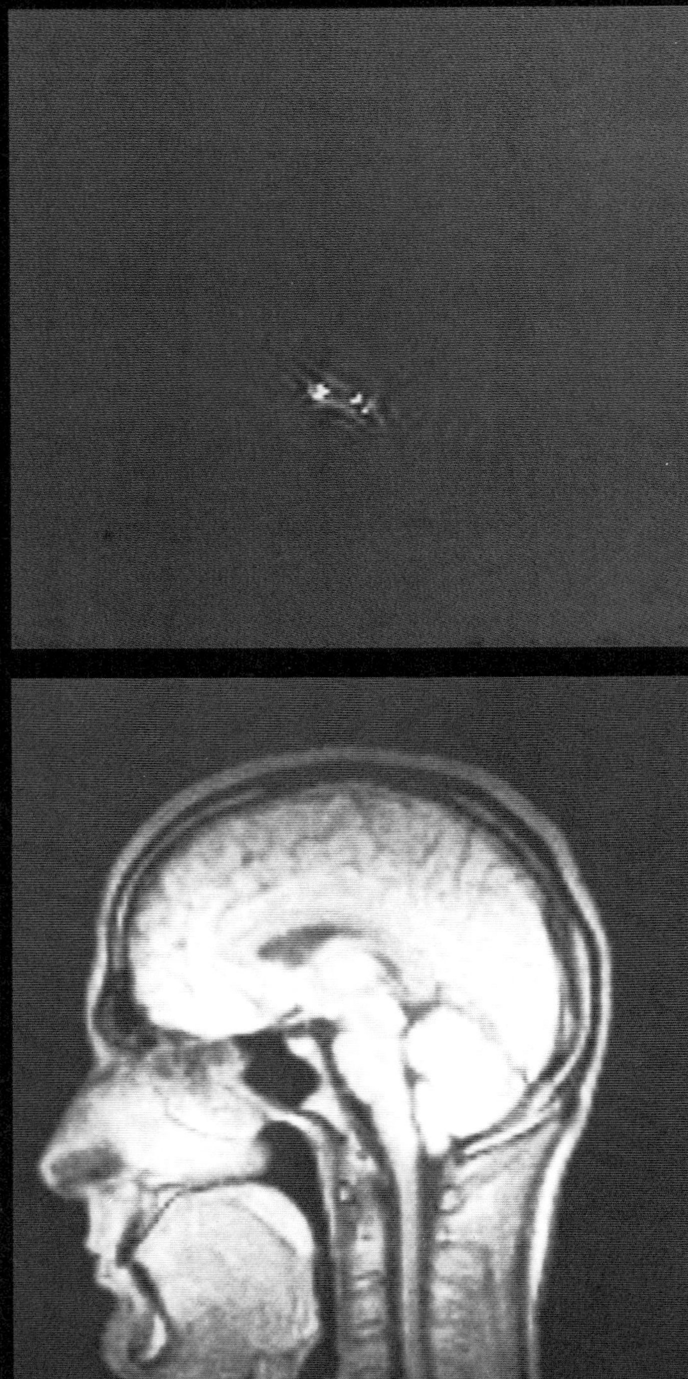

(a)

(b)

Fig. 4.9 *(a)* **Digitised NMR echoes positioned one on top of another producing a two-dimensional array which** *(b)* **then undergoes two-dimensional Fourier transform to produce an image**

In simultaneous slice acquisition the orientation of the sections, whether transverse, sagittal or coronal, must be determined prior to the start of acquisition. In the three main pulse sequences, the repetition time *TR* is of sufficient length to enable the nuclei to return, or return partially to their equilibrium position. In inversion recovery and spin echo sequences this pulse repetition time is of the order of 1 to 2 s. A similar value for *TR* is used in the saturation recovery sequence when largely proton density information is required. This means that during a large proportion of the pulse sequence time nothing is actually happening and we are simply waiting for the nuclei to return partially to equilibrium before the next RF pulse is applied. In simultaneous slice acquisition use is made of this period to excite and detect other slices without interfering with the section that is returning to equilibrium. This is illustrated in Fig. 4.10 using a saturation recovery sequence as an example. As can be seen there is a long delay between the NMR signals if a single slice is imaged. Imagine, however, that immediately after the first signal has been detected from section A, resonance is induced in section B by selective excitation. Remember that the position of a slice is selected by applying a particular frequency in conjunction with a magnetic field gradient. If the same magnetic field gradient is applied but a slightly different RF is used then a section adjacent to the previous section will resonate. After the signal from

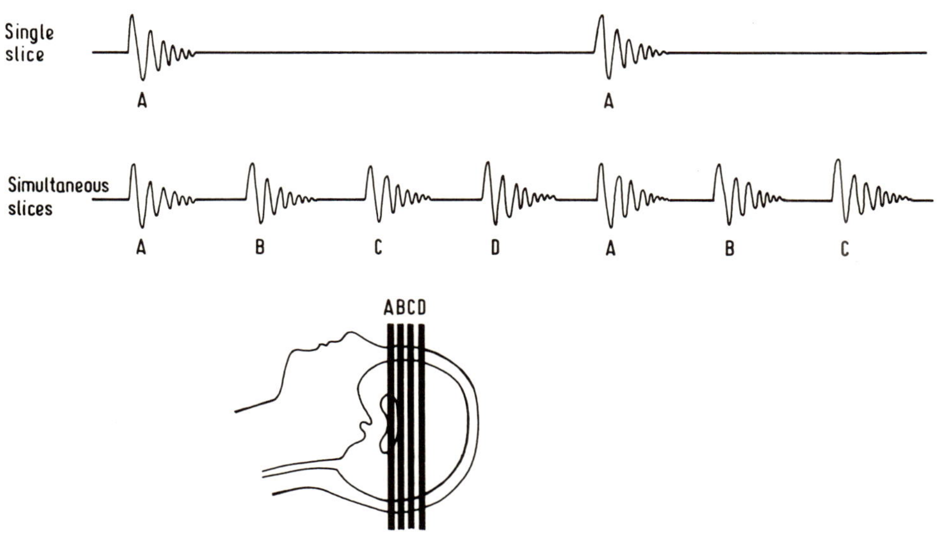

Fig. 4.10 Simultaneous slice acquisition with a saturation recovery pulse sequence. In single slice acquisition a signal is detected from slice A with an interval to allow a partial return to equilibrium. In simultaneous acquisition this period is used to obtain signals from slices B, C and D by applying different radiofrequencies which will not interfere with slice A

section B has been detected section C is caused to resonate by using a different frequency again. In the example given resonance is induced in four sections before an RF pulse at the original frequency is applied to produce resonance in slice A once more. Because the frequencies used for selective excitation are different for all the slices, nuclei in section A would not have been influenced in any way by the excitation of the other three slices and as a consequence will return towards the equilibrium position in exactly the same way as if the single section A was being acquired. Thus during simultaneous slice acquisition the acquisition time for a single slice is not decreased, but rather a number of slices are acquired in the same time that it would previously have taken to acquire a single slice.

In practice it is usual to leave a gap between the slices so acquired, as illustrated in Fig. 4.10, to prevent any interference occurring at the edges of the slices. This is because the slice profile is not perfectly square but has rounded edges and side lobes. Another simultaneous slice acquisition can then be performed to collect information from the sections in between. The images can be interleaved so that information is available from a complete volume within the patient. It is possible to acquire simultaneously 8, 16 or even 32 sections depending on the pulse sequence used and the timing of the pulse sequence parameters. Clearly the shorter the value of TR in any pulse sequence the fewer the number of sections that can be acquired.

Volume acquisition

Although simultaneous slice acquisition obtains data from a volume within a patient it is a planar imaging technique (*see* Fig. 4.1). Quite different from this is the technique of volume acquisition when each NMR signal comes not from a selected plane but from a much larger selected volume. Unlike simultaneous slice acquisition there is no necessity to preselect the orientation of the sections to be imaged. Volume acquisition produces a true three-dimensional representation of the patient from which a tomographic section at any orientation can be software-selected at the end of the acquisition.

Selective excitation is used to produce resonance in a volume in the patient by applying a much wider range of radiofrequencies than would usually be used to excite a single slice. The method of data reconstruction is an extension of 2DFT to three-dimensional Fourier transform. Spatial information in the x and z directions is encoded in the frequency and phase respectively as before and n_z different G_z phase encoded gradients are used. In volume acquisition the G_y gradient is not only used for selective excitation of the volume but also to phase encode spatial information in the y direction. The second phase encoding G_y gradient is applied at the same time as

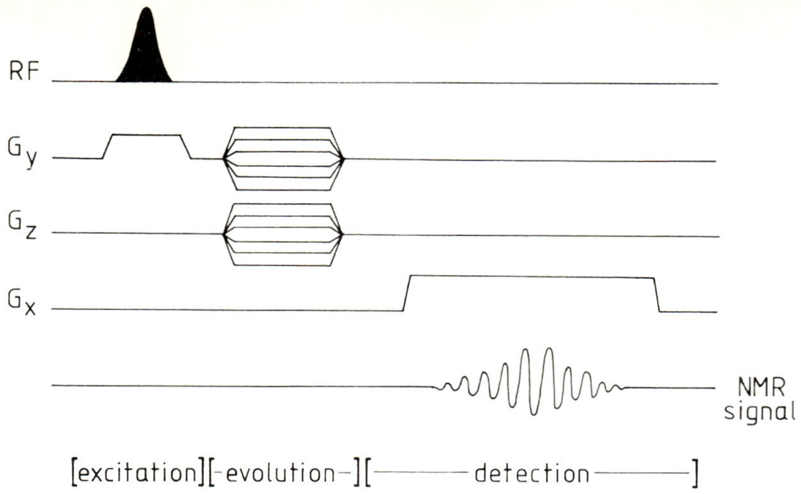

Fig. 4.11 RF and gradient pulse sequence for image production using three-dimensional Fourier transform (3DFT)

the G_z phase encoding gradient during the evolution period. To obtain spatial information in the third direction a number n_y of different phase encoding gradients must be used. For each particular G_y phase encoding gradient all n_z different G_z phase encoding gradients must be applied. As a consequence instead of n_z NMR signals being collected, as was the case with 2DFT, a much larger number $n_z \times n_y$ NMR signals need to be collected for a volume acquisition.

A typical RF and gradient sequence for volume acquisition is shown in Fig. 4.11. The advantage of volume acquisition is its ability to acquire all the data in a complete volume after which the operator can display any section at any orientation in any plane. However, the disadvantage is the longer time taken to image compared with simultaneous slice acquisition.

Real time MRI

One technique of MRI which is not as yet commercially available is that of echo planar imaging first proposed by Mansfield (1977). A section is selected using a gradient G_y together with a selective RF pulse. The FID of the section is then observed in a periodically switched gradient $\pm G_x$. Further information concerning the spatial distribution within the section is obtained by applying an additional steadily broadening gradient G_z during the signal sampling period. A complete image can be obtained in 40–60 ms, though the resolution obtained is much poorer than conventional MRI. This technique is currently in its development stage but may prove to be of clinical value in the future.

5

MRI equipment

The magnet

The largest item of hardware in an MRI system is the magnet which produces the constant external magnetic field. There are three types of magnet: resistive, superconducting and permanent. The choice of magnet is dependent on a variety of considerations but all must produce a stable uniform magnetic field throughout a slice or volume large enough to contain the appropriate region of the human body. The terms magnetic field uniformity or homogeneity are interchangeable and refer to the amount of variation in the magnetic field. It is not possible to manufacture a magnet with a perfectly uniform magnetic field: there is always some slight variation within, for example, a 40 cm diameter sphere. The homogeneity of a magnet is quoted in terms of parts per million (ppm) within a defined volume. For example, in a given volume the highest value could be 1.0001 T and the lowest 1.0000 T, resulting in a homogeneity of 100 ppm. The difference between the maximum and minimum field value is divided by the mean field value multiplied by 10^6. One word of caution when looking at figures of the homogeneity of an MRI magnet: sometimes the value is expressed as $\pm$ppm (in the example given 100 ppm would be the same as ± 50 ppm). In order to achieve good homogeneity for imaging purposes, electrical and sometimes mechanical adjustments must be made to the magnet gradually to improve the homogeneity. This process is known as shimming.

Resistive magnet

The first type of magnet which we will consider is the resistive magnet. When an electric current is passed through a loop of wire a magnetic field is generated as illustrated in Fig. 5.1. The magnetic field generated at the centre of the loop is perpendicular to the plane containing the current-carrying loop. A pair of such coils arranged adjacent to one another is known as a Helmholtz pair and produces a region of reasonable homogeneity at the centre between the two coils. In MRI a further two coils are used, one on either side of the central pair, a configuration which produces acceptable homogeneity over a sufficiently large volume (Fig. 5.2). The coils are constructed by winding thin bands of aluminium, of the order of

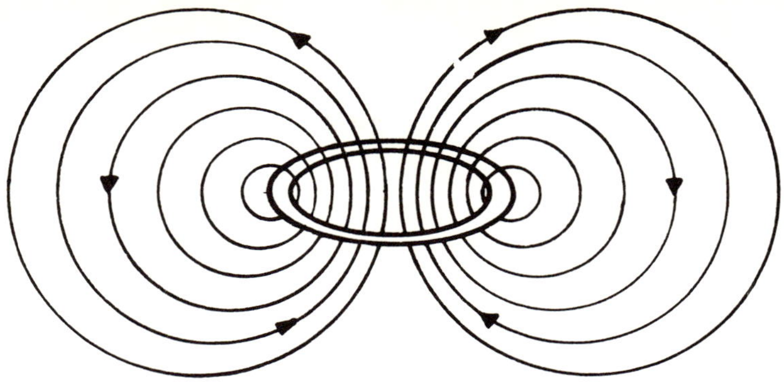

Fig. 5.1 Magnetic field from a horizontal loop of wire carrying an electric current; in the centre, the field is perpendicular to the plane containing the loop

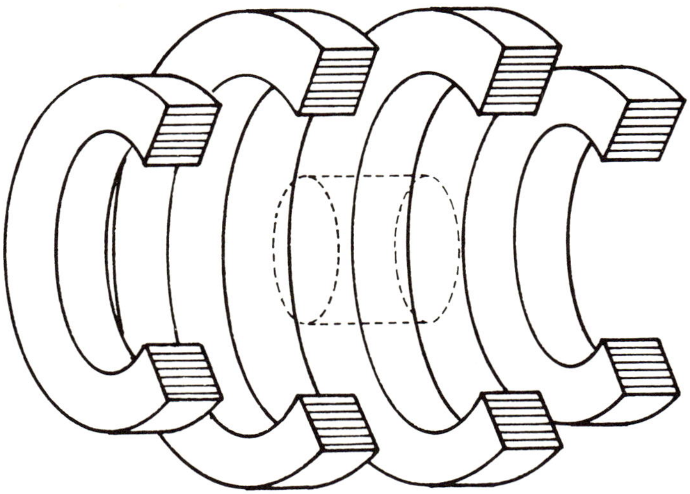

Fig. 5.2 Configuration of four vertically mounted coils in a resistive magnet which produce a region of high magnetic field homogeneity within the dotted region at the centre

2 mm thick, which are insulated from one another. The choice of aluminium is a compromise between the factors of weight, resistance and cost. Field strengths of up to 0.15 T are obtained using resistive magnets, the energy used to generate the field being dissipated as heat. A magnet with a field strength of 0.1 T uses approximately 30 kW of electricity. Water-cooling pipes are built within the rings of the magnet to dissipate this heat. Either mains water running to waste, or a closed loop refrigeration unit, can be used to supply cold water to the magnet.

The orientation of the ring magnets used in MRI systems can

be either vertical, as in Fig. 5.2, or horizontal with the result that the direction of the main magnetic field is either horizontal or vertical respectively. Most resistive magnets have a horizontal field so that the patient enters through the rings of the magnet. In a magnet with a vertical magnetic field the patient enters between the two central larger ring magnets. It has been suggested that this orientation has some advantages over the more usual horizontal field at lower field strengths because of the RF coil that can be used. A resistive magnet is shimmed by adjusting the relative position and orientation of the four magnets and by adjusting the position of much smaller shim coils within the magnet. Homogeneities of between 50 ppm and 200 ppm over a 45 cm diameter region are generally achieved using resistive magnets for MRI.

Superconducting magnets

Field strengths above 0.2 T are impractical using resistive magnets because of the dissipation of the heat and thermal instability. At field strengths above this superconducting magnets must be used. Superconducting (or cryogenic) magnets utilise the property that at very low temperatures electrical resistance is reduced to zero. In a resistive magnet heat is generated in overcoming the resistance of the conducting material within the coils; if the resistance is zero it therefore follows that heat dissipation will also be zero. Ring magnets, generally made from niobium–titanium alloy in a copper matrix, are enclosed and surrounded by liquid helium to lower the temperature of the windings to 4.2°K (−269°C) as shown in Fig. 5.3. This is then surrounded by a further layer of cooling material, this time liquid nitrogen at 77.4°K (−196°C), which is used to reduce the boil-off rate of the liquid helium, as it is more expensive than liquid nitrogen. At the temperature of liquid helium the windings of the coils have zero resistance, so if an electric current is applied and the source then removed it continues to circulate within the coil. Thus once an electric field is generated and the low temperature maintained, a constant stable magnetic field is present without the need for a continual supply of electricity. The saving in electricity is more than balanced by the cost of liquid helium and liquid nitrogen (referred to as cryogens) which continually boil-off and must be replaced at regular intervals. If for any reason, possibly due to a fault within the magnet, the resistance of a coil rises above zero the circulating electric current will immediately be dissipated as heat causing some of the cryogens to boil-off rapidly and the magnetic field to disappear. This process is known as 'quenching'.

Magnetic field strengths of between 0.15 T and 2.0 T have been generated by superconducting magnets and used for MRI. The

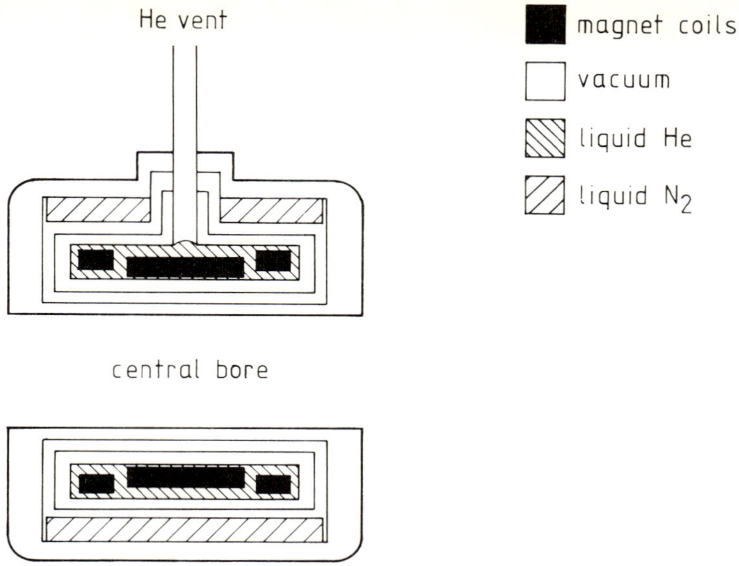

Fig. 5.3 Cross-section through a cryogenic magnet showing the magnet coils surrounded by liquid helium which in turn is kept at a low temperature by a combination of vacuum jackets and liquid nitrogen

magnets are shimmed electrically using an array of shim coils within the magnet. The process of shimming a superconducting magnet is far easier than shimming a resistive magnet and takes far less time. Typical homogeneities obtained from superconducting magnets are 10 ppm to 50 ppm over a 45 cm diameter region. Cryogenic magnets are also inherently more stable than resistive magnets because the circulating electric current is always constant, whereas in resistive magnets there can be some variation in the electrical power supply. The problem of variations in the power supply in resistive magnets can, however, be overcome by feedback devices.

Permanent magnets

Both resistive and superconducting magnets have appreciable running costs for electricity and cryogens respectively. The idea therefore of a permanent magnet for MRI is attractive because of the absence of such costs. Possible disadvantages are weight and thermal stability. A permanent magnet produced by one company has a field strength of 0.3 T and weighs 100 tonnes. It is claimed that the distribution of the magnet over a reasonably large area does not produce a major problem due to its weight. A further advantage is that the field around the magnet which will affect the surrounding environment is much lower than from a resistive magnet or superconducting magnet of comparable field strength.

Magnetic field strength

One question which has dominated MRI for the last couple of years is that of the optimum field strength for MRI. The advantages of the high and low field systems are listed in Table 5.1. The inherent spatial resolution of the system will improve as the field strength increases due to the improved signal-to-noise (S/N) ratio. Set against this is the fact that T_1 increases as the field strength increases and the separation between the T_1 values of different tissues decreases, resulting in a reduction in the contrast. The ability to detect abnormal pathology is a combination of both the contrast between the lesion and the surrounding tissue and the noise that is present on the image. Thus in MRI the contrast/noise ratio is often considered when comparing different field strength systems.

An additional advantage of MRI systems with field strengths above 1.5 T is that it may be possible to use them for NMR spectroscopy. However, it is our opinion that the role of MRI is such that any system purchased will very quickly be used full time for imaging purposes alone. In addition, spectroscopic examinations of patients are likely to be time-consuming. So though it may be technically possible to do both imaging and spectroscopy on the same system it is far better to have separate specialist NMR spectroscopic systems and MRI systems. The cost is almost always a factor in any consideration to purchase medical imaging equipment and there is considerable difference in cost between the high field and low field systems. Capital, installation and running costs are all significantly greater with the high field systems. In addition to the cost it is sometimes impossible to find a site in an older hospital for a high field system whereas a low field system, with or without magnetic shielding, can be installed.

One underlying problem in trying to find the optimum field strength for MRI is the fact that it may not even exist. There may in fact be no optimum field for MRI. In some clinical applications it may be more important to have high spatial resolution without tissue contrast whereas in others it may be more important to have acceptable spatial resolution but with high tissue contrast. So there may be as many 'optimum fields' as there are clinical applications for MRI.

Table 5.1 Relative advantages of low versus high field MRI systems

High field	*Low field*
Better spatial resolution May be used for NMR spectroscopy (> 1.5 T)	Better tissue contrast Cheaper to purchase, install and run

RF coils

It has been explained previously in Chapter 2 that resonance is induced in nuclei by the application of an oscillating magnetic field which must be both at a specific frequency and in a plane perpendicular to the direction of the main magnetic field. As in the case of the main magnetic field this oscillating magnetic field is produced by a loop of conducting material, the plane of which is perpendicular to the plane of the ring magnets producing the main magnetic field. The loop or loops of conducting material used to produce the oscillating magnetic field are referred to as the RF coil. There are two different types of RF coil used for clinical imaging depending on the orientation of the main magnetic field and these are illustrated in Fig. 5.4. As the transmission of the RF pulse and the reception of the NMR signal are carried out at different times it is possible for the same RF coil to be used as both transmitter and receiver: such a coil is sometimes referred to as a transceiver. However, there are some situations where there are advantages in using separate transmitter and receiver coils.

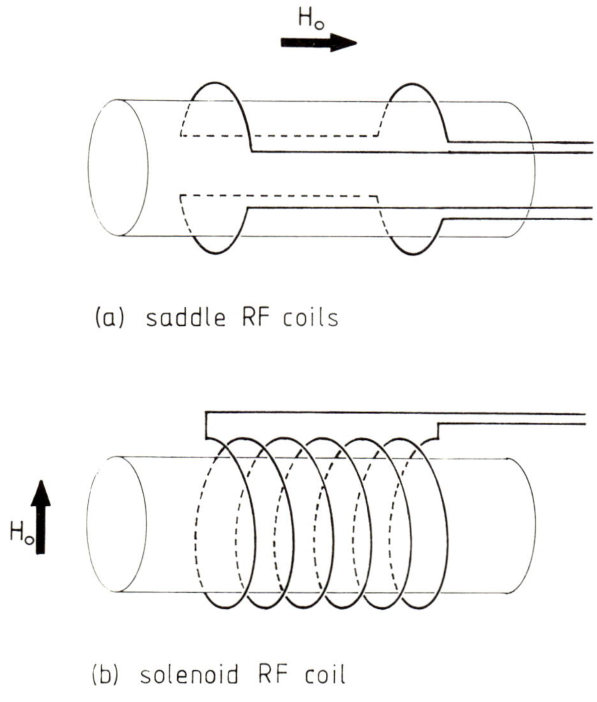

Fig. 5.4 Two main types of RF coils used for MRI with different orientations of H_o

MRI systems with vertically mounted ring magnets, producing the main magnetic field in the horizontal plane, use an RF coil known as a saddle coil (Fig. 5.4(*a*)). As the name suggests these RF coils are not simply circular loops of conducting material, but are contoured to fit more closely the shape of a patient. As the plane containing the ring magnets of the main field is the only plane which cannot contain an RF loop, the saddle coils can be placed above or below the patient or at either side. Using saddle coils it is possible for the coils in one plane to be used for transmission and the saddle coils in the perpendicular plane to be used as receiver. RF radiation used in MRI is at such a frequency that it tends to travel on the surface of any conductor used for the RF coil. Consequently the conducting material is usually a wide ribbon or tube of copper. In MRI systems which use saddle coils there is sometimes a selection of different coils available to fit the size of the patient.

When the main field is in the vertical direction and the plane of the main magnets is therefore horizontal a solenoid coil is generally used (Fig. 5.4(*b*)). With the vertical magnetic field one of the planes available for the RF coil is such that a circular coil can be used which surrounds the patient rather than being placed alongside as in the case of saddle coils. A solenoid RF coil is generally both a transmitter and receiver, being electronically switched between the two modes of operation.

There are a number of factors which must be considered in the design of the RF circuitry which will significantly influence various aspects of the final image. In order to obtain good NMR signal reception the quality factor (Q) of the RF coil must be as high as possible. The Q value is a measurement of energy lost in the RF coil and is defined as the signal frequency divided by the bandwidth at $\frac{1}{\sqrt{2}}$ of the peak amplitude. The electronics associated with the RF coil will influence not only the Q factor but also the surrounding environment. The presence of conducting loops, in particular in the same plane as the RF coil, will cause energy loss and hence lower the Q value. Any reduction in the Q value will reduce the signal-to-noise (S/N) ratio and consequently spatial resolution of the imaging system.

Both solenoid and saddle RF coils can be thought of as defining a volume, whether circular or elliptical, in cross-section. The proportion of this volume occupied by the sample is referred to as the RF coil 'filling factor'. In order to obtain a high sensitivity of signal detection it would seem reasonable that the filling factor should be as high as possible. This would be true if the sample to be measured did not alter the electrical properties of the RF coil in any way. However the human body is a conducting mass and if the RF coil is closely wrapped about the body, that is with a high filling factor, circulating currents will be induced which will absorb power from the coil. This will result in a lowering of the Q factor and hence reduction in S/N. Therefore in order to obtain a large S/N a compromise must be reached in finding the correct balance between filling factor and Q value.

When the RF radiation is transmitted through the patient it should ideally be uniformly distributed. Variations in the transmitted RF will result in the precessing angle being different in different parts of the section. Poor RF homogeneity could result in a supposed '90° pulse' producing resonance with precession angles of, for example, 80°, 90° or 100° in different parts of the tomographic section. Similar variations could also occur in a supposed 180° precession angle. Two factors affect the RF homogeneity within the patient: coil geometry and RF penetration. The use of the saddle design rather than a flat loop at the side of a patient improves the RF homogeneity. A solenoid RF coil is even better as it uniformly surrounds the patient. The best RF homogeneity is achieved when the diameter of the RF coil is large compared with the sample size. This is yet another compromise which must be considered in the design of suitable RF coils. The depth of penetration of the RF radiation decreases as a function of the square root of the frequency. In practice this is negligible for low field MRI systems and its importance at field strengths of around 1.5 T is a question of some debate. Early theoretical works suggested that at these field strengths RF penetration would be a significant problem but recent experiments carried out have demonstrated that NMR images can successfully be obtained.

The spatial resolution of images of a small part of the body near the surface can be improved using surface coils. These are simply circular loops of conductor which are of a size suitable for the region of interest and are placed on the surface of the patient. The body can be imaged with a high degree of spatial resolution to a depth approximately equal to the radius of the surface coil. Surface coils can be used to image regions of the body such as the eye, the spine or the breast.

RF pulses

The first RF pulse to be considered is the one which is most commonly used in MRI. The pulse consists of RF at the specific Larmor frequency contained with a Gaussian envelope. This is illustrated in Fig. 5.5(*a*); 90° pulses are of this type as are most 180° pulses, the latter however being of larger amplitude. The shape of the envelope of the pulse is specifically chosen to achieve good tomographic slice selection when used in conjunction with a selective gradient pulse; more recently sinc shaped pulses have been used to give squarer slice profiles. These 90° or 180° pulses can be used in all three standard pulse sequences: saturation recovery (*SR*), inversion recovery (*IR*) and spin echo (*SE*). One disadvantage of this type of 180° pulse is that it is not particularly suitable for precise quantitation of T_1. Any instability in the equipment or variations in RF homogeneity produces a 170° or 190° pulse instead of the ideal 180° pulse. Such variations have little effect on the qualitative assessment of the inversion recovery image, but significantly degrade the precision and accuracy of quantitative T_1 measurements. This can be overcome by performing a large number of inversion recovery sequences, each with a different *TI* value, to obtain more precise T_1 estimation; this method, however, is fairly time-consuming.

A second type of RF pulse is known as an adiabatic fast passage (AFP) and is illustrated in Fig. 5.5(*b*). Instead of being at a single frequency as in the previous case, a range of frequencies is swept through within the more rectangular envelope. This pulse is not slice-selective and effectively inverts the longitudinal component of magnetisation. As an inverting pulse it can be considered as a 180° pulse but only with respect to the direction of the equilibrium position. The AFP pulse is longer than a corresponding Gaussian 180° pulse, but requires less energy and a correspondingly lower power amplifier. The AFP pulse is not only very efficient at inverting the nuclei but does not require a specific power to produce inversion.

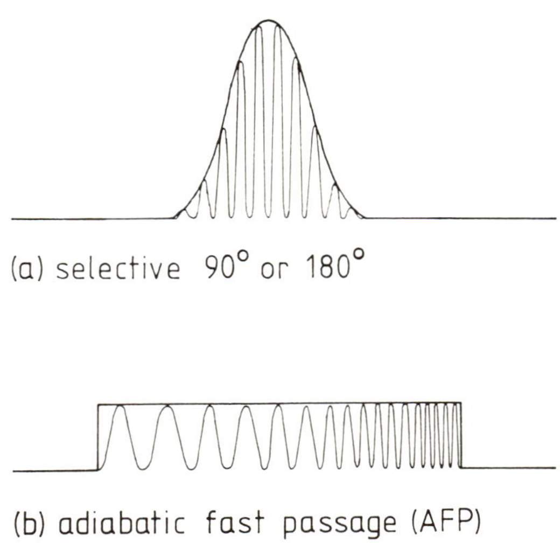

Fig. 5.5 *(a)* Gaussian shaped RF pulse, and *(b)* adiabatic fast passage (AFP) inverting RF pulse

If more power is applied than is actually needed the nuclei will not precess to 190°, 200° etc., they will simply remain inverted at 180°. As a consequence, if more than sufficient RF power is applied inversion can be achieved throughout the complete tomographic section regardless of slight variations in RF homogeneity. This pulse cannot be used for spin echo sequences but is ideal for use in inversion recovery when precise quantitative T_1 data is required.

Magnetic field gradients

It has been shown in the previous chapter that linear magnetic field gradients in all three coordinate directions are necessary for MRI. Although the amplitude of the three magnetic field gradients varies linearly in the three orthogonal coordinate directions the direction of the magnetic field in all three cases is parallel to the main magnetic field H_0. The magnetic field gradients are produced by circulating electric currents in loops of conducting materials of various geometries. The geometry of the gradient coils and the direction of the electric current will determine the orientation of the magnetic field gradient. The aim of gradient coil design is to produce magnetic gradients which vary in a linear fashion, the strength of the gradient being greater than any inhomogeneity of the main magnetic field. In general, there is a zero point at the centre of the gradient coil, the magnetic field produced being in the same direction as the external magnetic field on one side of the zero position and opposite to the direction of the main magnetic field on the other side of the zero position. The magnetic field experienced by the patient is the gradient field plus the main field as shown in Fig. 4.2. (p. 37).

Examples of three gradient coil configurations are illustrated in Fig. 5.6. The first and simplest is a Maxwell pair of coils with a current flowing in opposite directions Fig. 5.6(*a*). This produces a magnetic field gradient which will vary linearly in the z direction, G_z. The conductor configurations for generating field gradients G_x and G_y are more complex. The same design of conductor configuration can be used for both G_x and G_y, one being orientated at 90° to the other. The coil configuration used in early MRI systems to produce G_x and G_y gradients is illustrated in Fig. 5.6(*b*). The linear gradient field is generated by four appropriately spaced straight wires all with currents in the same direction. As it is only the straight wires nearest the centre of the magnet which produce the linear gradient, the four coils making up this gradient configuration must be sufficiently large so that the field from other parts of the coil does not interfere. In the example in Fig. 5.6.(*b*) the four coils produce a gradient G_x. A further four coils at 90° to these would be needed

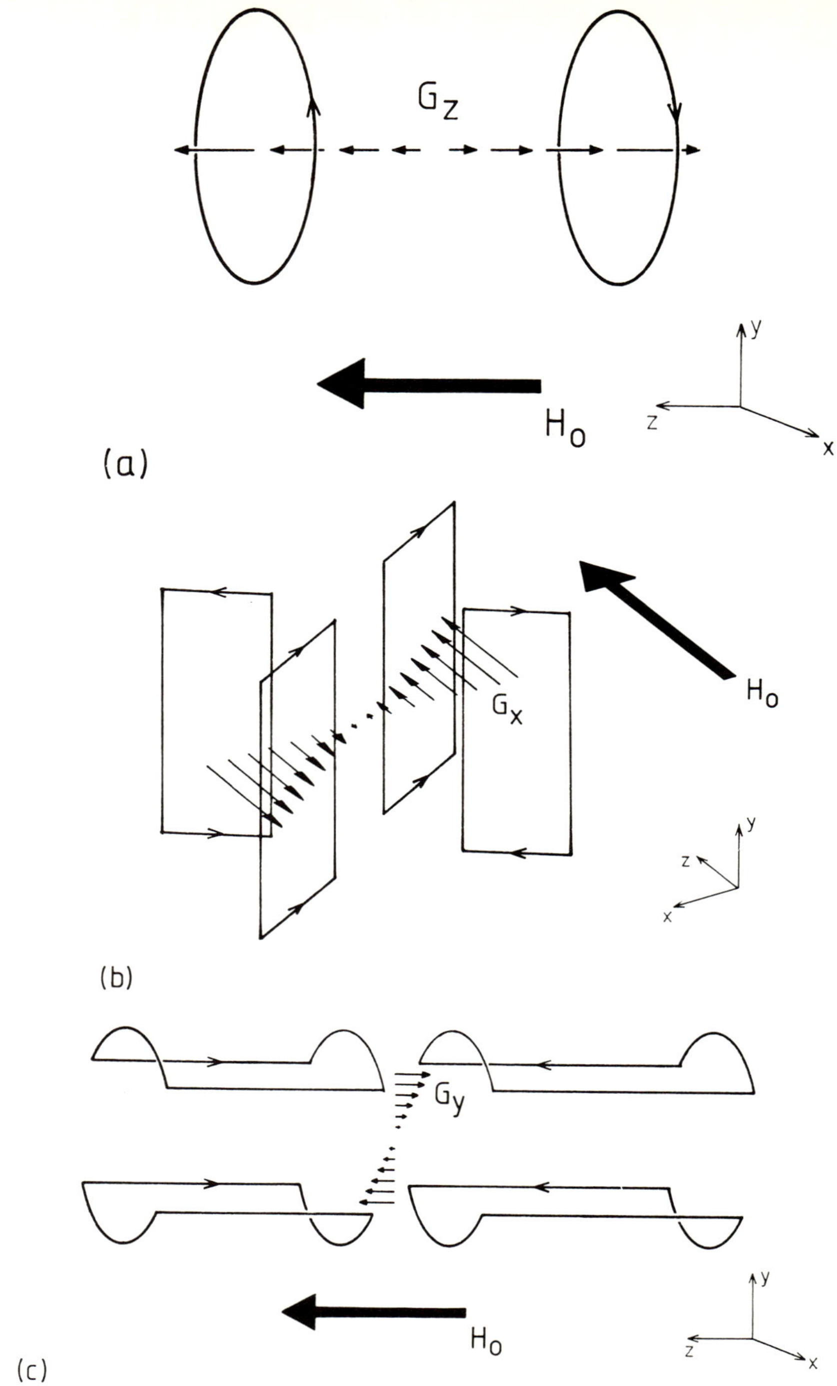

Fig. 5.6 Gradient coil configurations producing linear gradients: *(a)* Maxwell pair producing G_z; *(b)* straight wire configuration producing G_x; and *(c)* Golay coils producing G_y

for the G_y gradients. The third example in Fig. 5.6(*c*) is more commonly used now in MRI systems and is known as the Golay configuration. These gradient coils can be wrapped around the cylinder which surrounds the patient inside the imager. The magnetic gradient generated by these coils will be linear for a distance of just under three-quarters of the radius from the central position.

The variation in magnetic field produced by a gradient is approximately two orders of magnitude lower than the main magnetic field. For example in a 0.3 T system the magnetic field gradient may vary from −1.5 mT to +1.5 mT across the volume or section to be imaged, usually 30–40 cm. This corresponds to a magnetic field gradient of 10 mT/m, the unit in which magnetic gradients are usually expressed.

Computer

The computer hardware required for MRI is in general not significantly any more complex than the computers used for other imaging techniques such as X-ray CT. The computer is used to control the timing of the pulse sequences, sending out signals which drive the RF amplifier and the three gradient amplifiers; not only the timing but also the shape of the RF and gradient pulses can be computer-controlled. The NMR signal which is generated will be fed back into the computer and digitised using analogue-to-digital convertors (ADCs). This process is illustrated in Fig. 5.7. The NMR signal which is fed into the computer will be in analogue form, that is

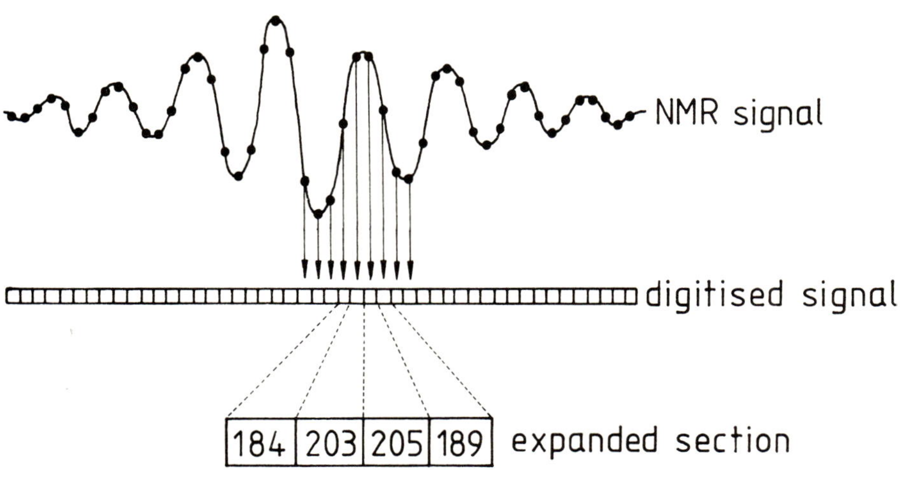

Fig. 5.7 Analogue-to-digital conversion of an NMR signal. The continually varying signal is sampled at sufficiently close intervals and the voltage detected is converted to a number which can be stored in the computer

a voltage which is continually varying in time. This continually varying voltage is sampled at fixed time intervals and stored as numerical data. If the interval between sampling is too long then the numerical representation of the signal will be inaccurate. Figure 5.8 demonstrates the effect that sampling too infrequently would have on the stored representation of the original NMR signal. The NMR signal is generally digitised into 128, 256, 512 or 1024 values. These numbers are all factors of two (2^7–2^{10}) and are used because they are mathematically and computationally convenient. In the construction of an NMR image a large number of signals are used; as each signal enters the computer it is digitised until at the end of a scan an array of data will be present consisting of many lines of digitised NMR signals stored one on top of the other. Such an array of data is referred to as a matrix. The computer will then be used to perform a two-dimensional Fourier transform on this data (see Chapter 4) to produce an image which is made up of 128 × 128, 256 × 256 or 512 × 512 elements. These elements of this matrix are known as pixels, an abbreviation of picture cells. The image can then be displayed on a monitor, the intensity on the screen being directly related to the number in the image matrix.

Although the NMR image may be stored in for example, a 128 × 128 matrix it can be displayed on a larger 256 × 256 matrix. In such a situation the image is said to be interpolated. Each pixel of the original matrix will be divided into four, the value of each of these smaller pixels being a function both of the original larger pixel value and the value of its immediately neighbouring pixels. Such an image can be more pleasing to the eye but does not in fact contain any extra spatial information. When considering NMR images, particularly in terms of resolution and array size it is important to note whether the image displayed on a monitor has been interpolated or not.

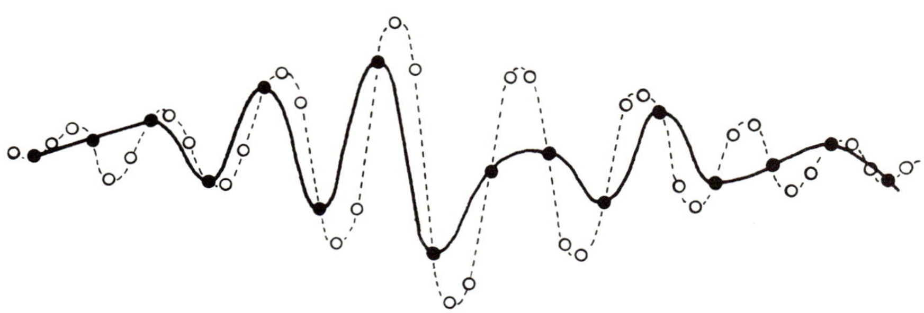

Fig. 5.8 The signal considered in Fig. 5.7 (dotted line) has been sampled too infrequently, the sampling interval being three times longer than before; the closed circles correspond to the positions of sampling and the distorted representation of the signal obtained from the sampling points (solid line) can clearly be seen

MRI systems

Vertical cross-sections through MRI systems with the two different field orientations are illustrated in Fig. 5.9. The mode of entry for the subject is clearly seen as are the gradient and RF coils. All MRI systems are surrounded by an RF shield, usually aluminium sheet,

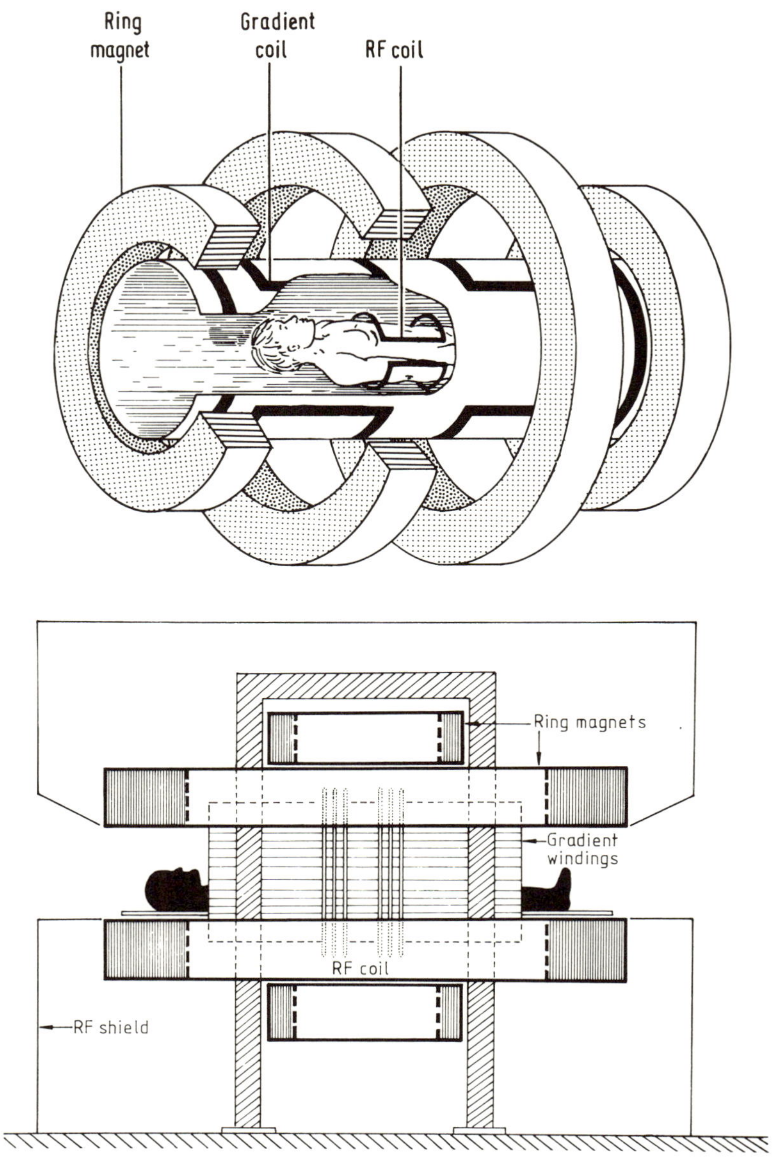

(a)

(b)

Fig. 5.9 *(a)* Cross-section through an MRI system with the ring magnets mounted in the vertical direction and the magnetic field horizontal. *(b)* Cross-section through a system with horizontally orientated ring magnets and a vertical magnetic field (Hutchison and Smith, 1983).

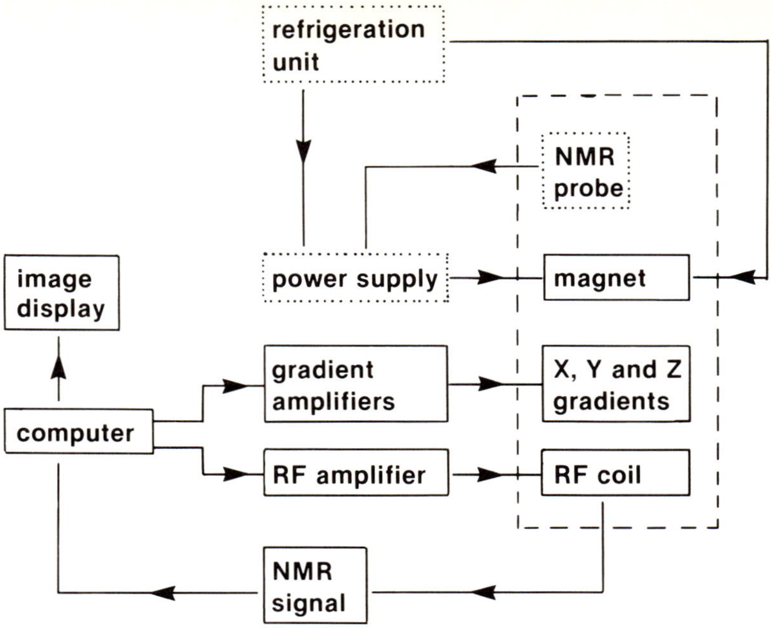

Fig. 5.10 Block diagram of the basic components of an MRI system; in a cryogenic magnet the power supply and NMR probe would not be present

to reduce interference. A block diagram of the components of an MRI system is shown in Fig. 5.10. The components are similar for a resistive and a cryogenic system, the power supply and NMR feedback device being absent in the latter.

Signal-to-noise ratio

In all imaging techniques there is an element of noise, which is random, which will degrade the information available from the signal in which we are interested. With ionising radiation there is a random element of noise which is a function of the signal size itself. Because of this interdependence, and also because the signal itself is relatively large, the concept of the signal-to-noise ratio is not a particularly major factor in designing such imaging equipment. For MRI, however, this is not the case; the signal is relatively small and the noise is independent of the signal size. The signal-to-noise ratio, or S/N as it is often referred to, of MRI significantly influences the spatial resolution of the image. An example of an NMR signal with good and poor S/N is illustrated in Fig. 5.11. To obtain good spatial resolution it must be possible to detect very small differences in frequency of the NMR signal. Any noise that is present in the signal will be at relatively high frequencies which makes the detec-

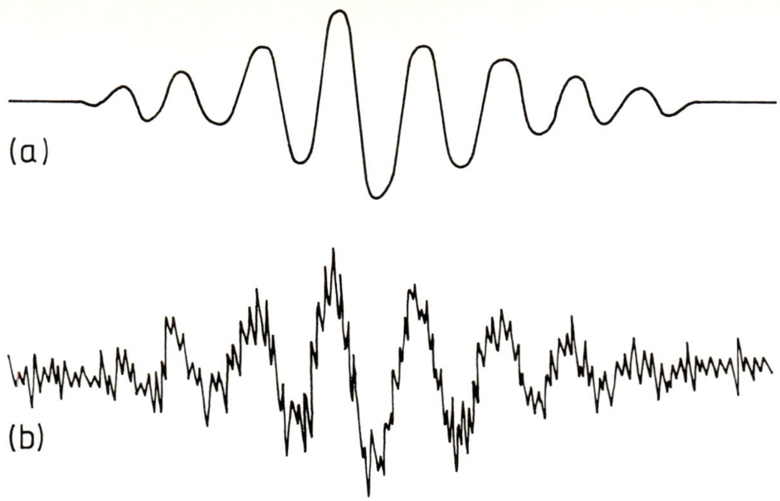

Fig. 5.11 NMR signal with *(a)* good S/N, and *(b)* poor S/N

tion of small frequency differences within the signal more difficult and hence the spatial resolution is degraded. The presence of noise on the signal also increases the background in an NMR image. An example of an NMR image with good and poor S/N is illustrated in Fig. 5.12.

Although the S/N of a single NMR signal obtained from an imager influences the S/N in the final image, the instrument S/N is not necessarily equivalent to the image S/N. There are various factors which influence the former and additional factors which can influence the latter. The main design criteria for many MRI systems is to obtain a high S/N within a time that is practical for patient investigation. One word of caution; although spatial resolution is important in MRI, it is possible to achieve a high S/N at the expense of T_1 contrast.

The S/N increases as the frequency of resonance and consequently magnetic field strength increases. This has been one of the main factors in the decision that some companies have made to move to high magnetic field strengths such as 1.5 T for imaging purposes. Depending on various initial assumptions the theoretical S/N will increase as a function of frequency to the power of 7/4 or 3/2. However, in practice this relationship becomes linear in MRI systems with a high magnetic field.

The range of frequencies that are used to encode spatial information and which the imager is set up to detect, known as the bandwidth, will influence S/N. Clearly the wider the bandwidth $\Delta\omega$ the greater the amount of RF noise that will be detected. The bandwidth chosen is influenced by the size of the magnetic field gradient, which

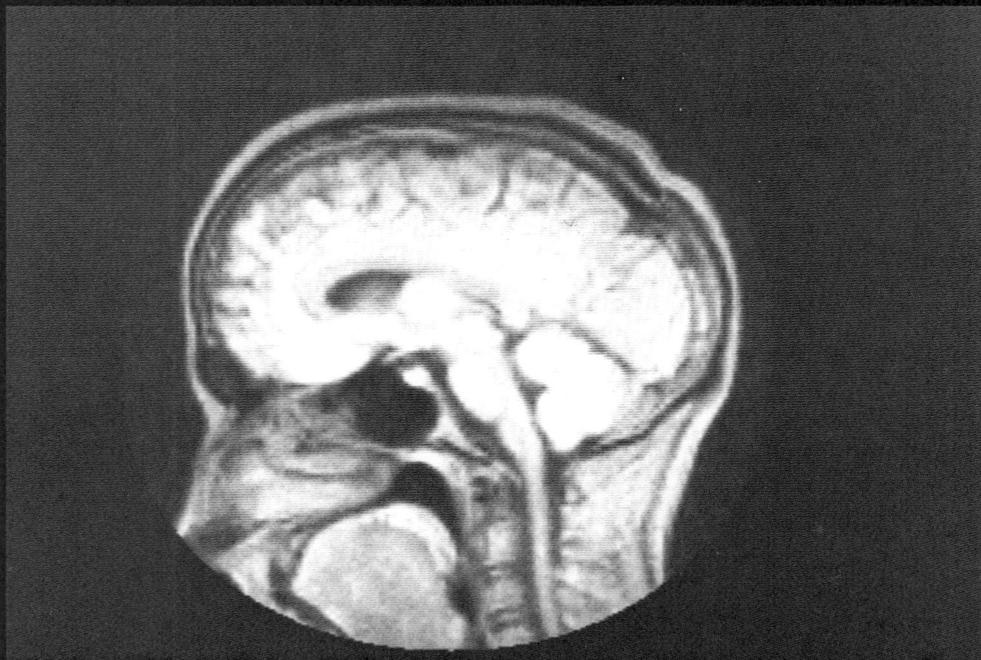

(a)

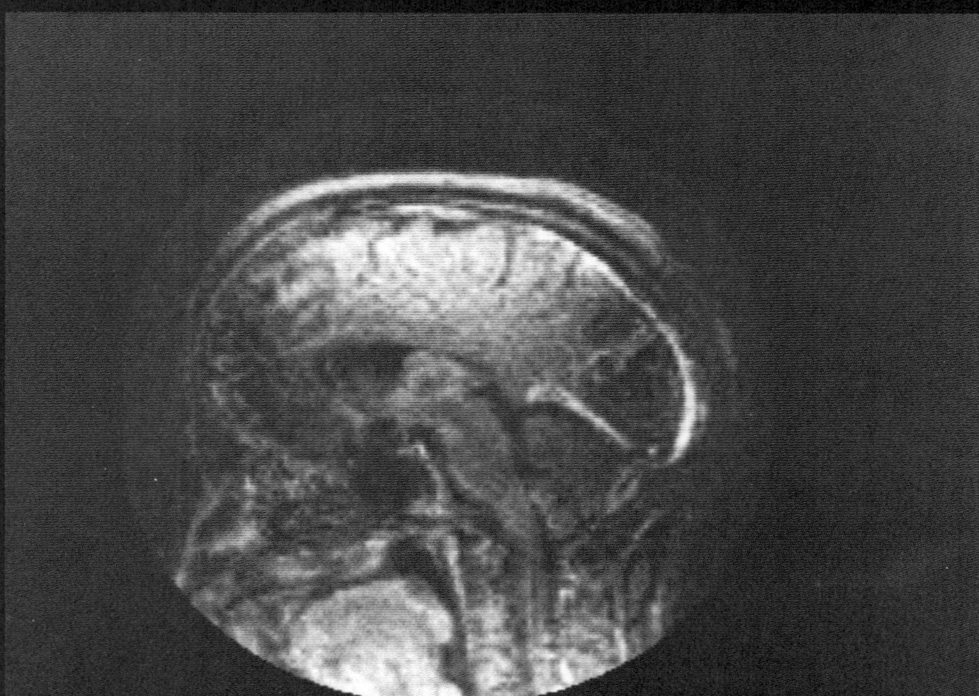

(b)

Fig. 5.12 Image with *(a)* good S/N, and *(b)* poor S/N. The poor S/N in *(b)* was obtained by reducing the NMR signal size but keeping the noise constant

determines the range of frequencies; this in turn is determined by the overall homogeneity of the main magnetic field. Better homogeneity will result in lower magnetic field gradients which in turn will result in a reduced bandwidth. S/N will vary as a function of $\frac{1}{\sqrt{\Delta\omega}}$.

The volume of the sample from which the signal is obtained influences S/N; the larger the volume the larger the signal and hence the larger the value of S/N. This is most apparent in planar imaging where the section width will influence S/N, the wider the section the better the S/N. However, if the section becomes too wide, although the S/N is increased the spatial resolution is decreased because of partial volume effect.

The design of the RF coil will influence S/N. At lower magnetic field strengths a solenoid RF coil has an increased S/N compared with a saddle coil by a factor of 2 to 3.

All the variables discussed so far influence the S/N of the NMR signal. However an image is obtained from a number of NMR signals, the S/N of the final image being related to the number of signals collected which determines the total time taken to obtain an image. If an image is constructed from n NMR signals, the final signal value in the image will be a function of n whereas the noise, because of its random nature will be a function of $\sqrt{n}$. The S/N of an NMR image will therefore increase as the square root of the number of NMR signals and hence the square root of the time taken. If the imaging time is doubled there will therefore be a $\sqrt{2}$ improvement in S/N. When comparing images from various MRI systems it is therefore important to note the time taken to acquire the image as good S/N can be obtained by collecting an image for a long period of time. Long acquisition times are impractical because of patient movement and because of the need for high patient throughput. As a consequence a compromise must be reached between S/N and imaging time.

Environmental considerations

Prior to the installation of an MRI system it is important to consider not only what effect the imager will have on its surrounding environment, but also what effect the surrounding environment can have on the performance of the imager. The magnetic field from the main magnet will extend a significant distance from the imager itself, the distance and strength of the field being a function of the main magnetic field strength. The field outside the MRI imager is referred to as the fringe field, and contours of magnetic field are circular

Table 5.2 Distance (in metres) of the fringe magnetic field strength from MRI systems with magnetic field values ranging from 0.08–1.5 T

			Magnet field strength (T)				
			0.08	0.15	0.3	0.5	1.5
Devices affected by MRI systems	Objects affecting MRI systems	Fringe magnetic field strength	*Distance from Magnet* (m)				
Cathode ray tubes X-ray tubes MRI computer Magnetic tape and discs Credit cards Analogue watches	Large static ferromagnetic objects	1 mT	3.8	4.9	6.2	7.4	10.6
Cardiac pacemakers		500 μT (5G)	4.6	6.0	7.5	9.0	12.9
	Large moving ferromagnetic objects, such as cars, lifts, etc. Power transformers	250 μT	5.8	7.6	9.4	11.3	16.2
Gamma cameras Image intensifiers CT scanners Photomultipliers Ultrasound systems		100 μT	7.9	10.3	12.9	15.5	22.1

in shape in the same plane as the ring magnets and elliptical in shape in the perpendicular direction extending further in the latter. The fringe field can interfere with other electrical equipment, such as electron microscopes or gamma cameras, and particular care must be taken with the possible effect on patients wearing cardiac pacemakers.

In the immediate environment of an MRI system static ferromagnetic material can limit the homogeneity that can be achieved in the magnet. Moving ferromagnetic material, such as lifts or cars can seriously interfere with the imager and so should be as far away as possible. An alternative, however, is to surround the magnet with large ferromagnetic sheets which will act as a magnetic shield though this can increase the cost of the imager, and the increase in weight can pose additional problems in the installation.

The other source of interference which will affect the MRI system is external RF radiation. The imager itself is usually surrounded by an RF shield consisting of aluminium sheets, but sometimes the complete room containing the NMR system has to be RF shielded. If there is interference at a specific frequency which interferes with the imager it is possible to change slightly the field strength of the main magnet and hence move the resonant frequency to a region where there is no such interference.

Approximate fringe field values and corresponding distances for various magnetic field strengths are listed in Table 5.2 with specific things which may affect or be affected by the MRI system.

6

Practical aspects of clinical imaging

Patient preparation

MRI is associated with some hazards, some of which are unique to the technique but of which one must be constantly aware. Magnetic fields cause hazards which can be divided into three types.

Nuisance

Credit cards can be erased if a person strays too close to the magnet; magnetic tapes such as in dictaphones and floppy discs will be erased; analogue watches may become magnetised and cease to work.

Projectile

Pieces of ferromagnetic matter too close to the magnet may be attracted into it with a considerable velocity. Persons going close to the magnet must therefore be screened for potentially dangerous objects which some people may be carrying such as screwdrivers or scissors. This hazard is negligible with low field strength systems (<0.1 T) but considerable with the high field systems.

Patient

Pacemakers These may be affected by the electrical fields generated during imaging particularly from the gradient fields. These may cause problems in the pacing unit giving rise to false pacing signals. This is an obvious and easily avoidable hazard and nobody with a pacemaker should be allowed near the magnet.

Aneurysm clips Any patient with a history of surgery on an intracranial aneurysm must be very carefully considered before being examined by MRI. Many of the clips used in clipping these aneurysms are ferromagnetic and move in a magnetic field. This movement will take the form of an applied torque on the clip as the patient is being inserted into the magnet and is subjected to the changing lines of magnetic flux. This hazard is therefore very important and real. It has been suggested that where possible neurosurgeons should use non-ferromagnetic clips to decrease the risk of clip detachment in subsequent MRI examinations. However, it would appear safer to suggest that any patient with an intracranial aneurysm clip should not be subjected to MRI. It is also true that the risk of detachment of these clips increases with the magnitude of the static field employed. Most other types of clips used in intracranial surgery such as the commonly used LIGA haemostatic clip are non-ferromagnetic and do not constitute a contraindication to MRI.

Other metallic objects The patient must also be closely examined for *metallic objects* on their person. Things which may be overlooked include small hairgrips and hearing aids behind the ear. If these are missed then not only is the image ruined in the region of the metal but there is a chance that the metallic object may become detached and be a dangerous projectile or may even get lost in the imager. There is a theoretical risk that if this happens the magnet may have to be shut down to retrieve it and this would obviously be very costly in terms of both time and money, particularly with a cryogenic system. Most jewellery is non-ferromagnetic and should not cause any problems, but it is safer to insist that all jewellery be removed before entering the imaging suite. It is not necessary to completely undress the patient when imaging the head but the top of zippers on dresses may cause artefacts especially on sagittal sections and these should be pulled down out of the region of interest. Full sets of dentures do not normally contain metal and therefore should pose no problems, but partial dentures frequently contain significant amounts of metal which results in serious degradation of the image in the region of the dental plate. Some other dental procedures such as 'crowns' also involve implanting a little metal in the mouth and this may also degrade the image.

Patients with epilepsy or cardiac arrhythmias

It is nowadays considered safe to image patients with a history of epilepsy or cardiac arrhythmias. It must be remembered, however, that the patient will be going into a confined space with restricted access and limited observation facilities. Medical and radiographic personnel should always be extra careful with those patients in whom there may be an increased risk of trouble such as an epileptic fit or loss of consciousness. Dyspnoeic patients may find the enclosed space inside the imager claustrophobic and it may be that the examination of such patients should be split up into short imaging sessions, bringing the patient out between each one for a rest. It should also be remembered that the examination may be quite protracted and this may prove difficult for some patients with poor bladder control. All MR imagers are safe from the electrical risks of flooding and therefore there would be no risk to the patient if he or she were incontinent. However, for the patient's comfort it is wise to enquire about such happenings in the elderly and ensure that the bladder is completely empty before starting the examination. Putting the patient on an incontinence sheet is also wise if there is a significant risk. This is also to be recommended when imaging paediatric patients where wetting is a constant risk.

Contrast agents

With regard to contrast agents little, if any, preparation is required in most MRI examinations. Even the contrast agents which may be used in the future do not appear to be associated with the side-effects of nausea and vomiting that are a feature of the iodinated contrast materials used in CT. Therefore, no specific instructions are required to be given to patients before attending for imaging. In the pelvis, however, it may be useful to ask the patient not to empty the bladder before the examination, in other words, to have a comfortably full bladder in order that one can use the long relaxation time urine as an anatomical landmark in the pelvis. Some workers have used simple contrast agents such as ferric chloride in the stomach and fatty compounds (milk, ice cream) in the small bowel but as yet there is no satisfactory or reproducible material for providing 'magnetic' bowel labelling. Several groups are working on this problem and there may soon be an oral agent available to 'outline' the bowel.

Setting up

This is less of a problem when compared with CT for several reasons. MRI allows for transverse, sagittal and coronal imaging with equal ease, unlike CT where planes other than the transverse are reformatted only after obtaining many thin contiguous transverse sections or, in the case of coronal orbital images, by maintaining the head in a position of hyperextension during scans. This routine acquisition of multiplanar sections means that we do not have to rely on accurately positioned transverse sections for localisation of any detected pathology, since the exact position of lesions can be so much more accurately localised by using all three planes. However, it is sound radiographic practice to adhere to a standard whenever possible since this will allow for easy comparison in follow-up examinations, and also permits rapid assessment of any change in size of pathology to be observed. Thus, it is useful to adopt a standard routine for each examination using standard radiographic principles and surface markings such as the orbitomeatal line in transverse head images. In particular anatomical situations it may be useful to slightly alter the plane of section. When obtaining coronal images of the brain stem it is useful to tilt the orbitomeatal baseline relative to the plane of section to avoid obtaining an oblique section. Movement of the head relative to the imaging plane is also useful when imaging the optic nerves in the sagittal plane when the side of interest can be tilted towards the midline so as to bring the nerve more parallel to the plane of section.

In a similar fashion to CT positioning is usually achieved using light sources and the head is normally positioned with the baseline parallel to the imaging plane in the transverse plane. Coronal and sagittal views can be selected by referring to the transverse image but in some situations it may be wise to commence with a sagittal image, for example, if the clinical signs point to a lesion of the brain stem or craniovertebral junction. Once the patient has been aligned he is then moved into the imager. This may be by a motor-driven couch system or the couch may simply be pushed into the system manually. Some people prefer to be pushed in since being transported into an enclosed space on a motor-driven system may give the impression of a crematorium! Once the patient is inside the imager slice selection is usually achieved electronically, and therefore involves no patient movement; some other systems rely on carefully controlled couch movement to change the position of the slice in a manner analogous to CT.

Claustrophobia

It is at the moment of entering the magnet that most patients experience claustrophobia. Many patients can be persuaded to continue but will require constant reassurance and surveillance during the remainder of the procedure. Sedation (diazepam, for example) may be a help, but most often a technique of gentle persuasion is the best policy. The rejection rate varies from centre to centre and also varies with the experience of the operators but can be expected to be less than 2%. If a multiple slice capability is available it should be used whenever possible. If one is looking for pathology without very definite clinical localising signs multiple transverse sections can be used as the initial investigation, and then any suspicious areas re-examined using a different pulse sequence. If any pathology is detected it can then be more accurately localised by using the other two planes. In some instances, however, where the clinical suspicion indicates a more localised lesion such as the cerebellopontine angle, it may be wiser not to employ the multiple slice capability and instead perform more averaging to improve the signal-to-noise and spatial resolution. The particular pulse sequence required will vary with the clinical problem as will be outlined in subsequent chapters.

Anaesthetics

Most adults and many children can be successfully examined with some tact, persuasion and perhaps a little sedation. However, most young children and some ill or confused adults may, as in CT, require a general anaesthetic before they can be successfully imaged. General anaesthetics can be administered during an MR examination but there are problems and, in general, these become greater as the field strength increases. As the magnitude of the static field increases so does the effect of nearby metal on the imager and the resultant image. Objects such as anaesthetic trolleys and gas cylinders will interfere with the quality of the field and may render useful imaging impossible; the projectile risk from such objects also increases with field strength. To keep these effects to a minimum ferromagnetic objects must be kept as far away from the imager as possible. This creates real problems for the anaesthetist since the lengths of tubing required to connect the patient to a gas source become very long, and also the anaesthetist may have to stay at a distance from the patient which does not allow for adequate supervision of an anaesthetised subject. For these reasons it is probably wise to suggest restricting general anaesthetics in MRI to the lower field strength systems (0.08–0.35 T). As well as the problem of administering the anaesthetic and the difficulty of supervision, the anaesthetist must also be told not to use any ferromagnetic materials in gas connections or endotracheal tubes. Patient monitoring can be easily achieved using the types of ECG leads used in cardiac gating procedures; respiratory monitoring can be accomplished using either non-metallic stethoscopes taped to the chest or by using an oesophageal stethoscope. A simple pulse monitor may be useful in some other patients that are perhaps ill or frail and this can be achieved by using a simple LED device which is secured round a finger and connected to a battery operated monitor.

Image artefacts

It has been stated previously in Chapter 3 that the intensity of any portion of the image in a given pulse sequence depends on the proton density, T_1 and T_2 of the tissue. This is true in static tissue but where there is rapid movement, such as blood flow, the signal intensity will also be influenced by the velocity. In short *TR* sequences, where there is only a partial return to equilibrium, blood outside the section of interest at equilibrium will move into the section and will result in a much larger signal than surrounding tissue. If the blood is flowing very rapidly then the blood will move out of the section in the time between the excitation and detection of the signal causing a complete lack of signal on the image. Thus flowing blood can produce what is known as a paradoxical enhancement (Fig. 6.1(*a*)), where the intensity of the signal gradually increases as the velocity increases up to a maximum value. As the velocity increases further the signal will decrease until no signal is received. The flow effect can be influenced by changing the pulse sequence, and can be useful in separating different structures in regions such as the mediastinum. Research is being carried out in several centres to use the effect of velocity on the NMR signal to quantitate blood flow in regions of the body that cannot be measured by more conventional techniques such as Doppler ultrasound.

Patient movement does not simply cause blurring of the images but results in aliasing in the phase-encoded axis of the image. The effect of cardiac motion is illustrated in Fig. 6.1(*b*) and patient movement in Fig. 6.1(*c*).

Metallic objects can either cause a small localised loss of signal (Fig. 6.1(*d*)) or a more general disruption of the field homogeneity resulting in a overall poorer quality noise image due to a poorer signal-to-noise ratio (Fig. 6.1(*e*)).

In the two-dimensional Fourier transform method of image production there can sometimes be an artefact directly in the centre of the image. An example of a Fourier transform artefact is illustrated in Fig. 6.1(*f*). If there is a very small region of high signal in a patient that occurs in the centre of the image it is advisable to repeat the section so that the region is away from the centre.

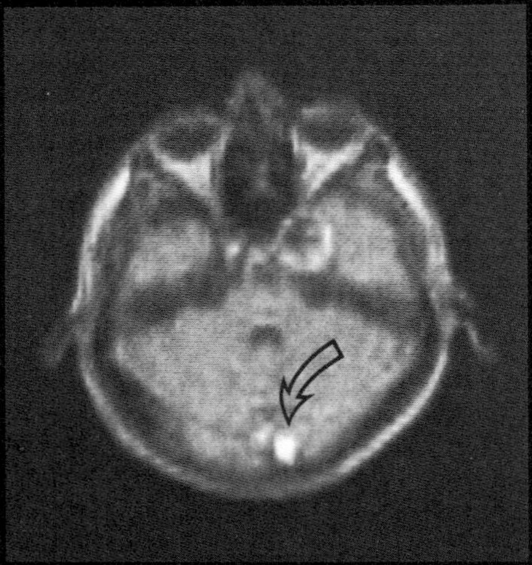

(a)

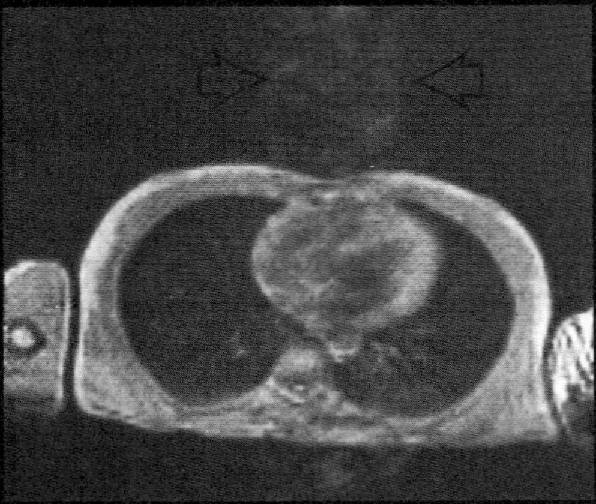

(b)

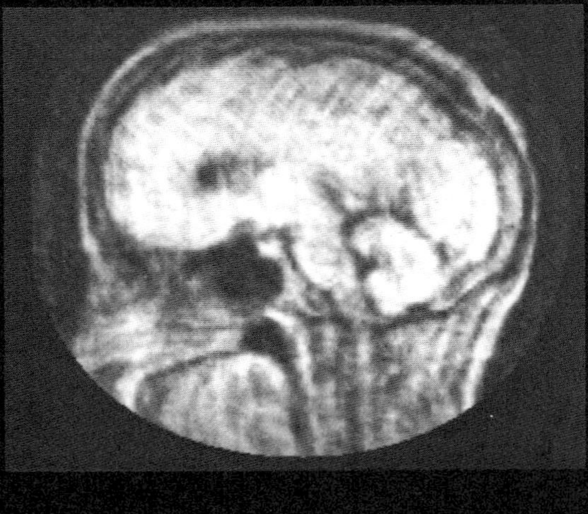

(c)

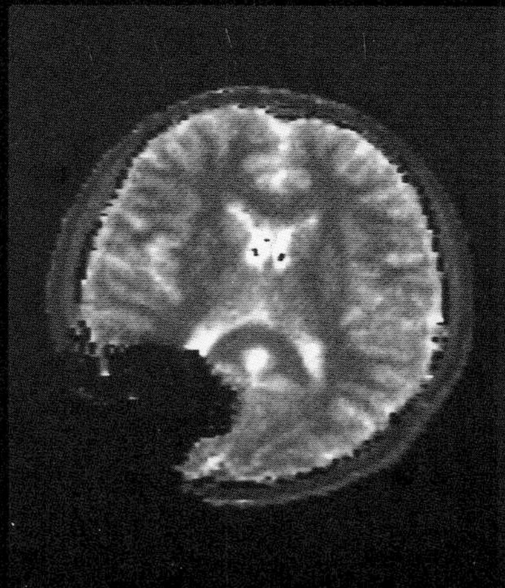

(d)

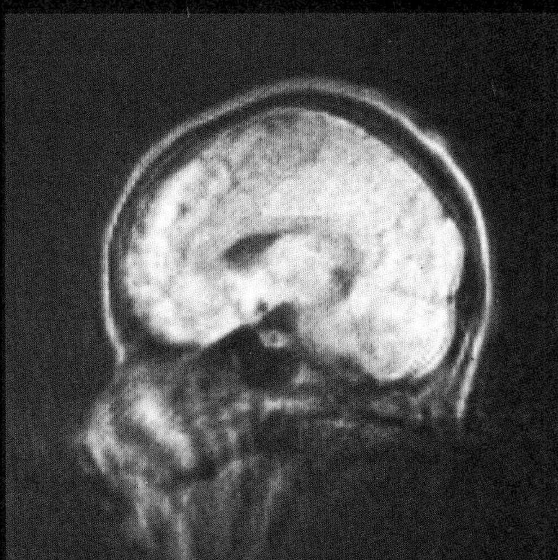

(e)

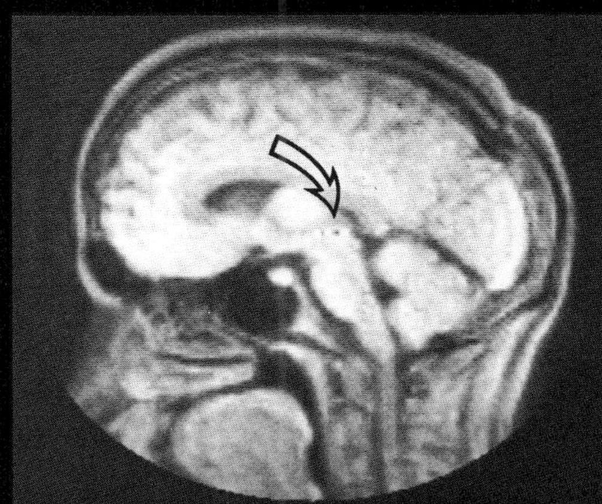

(f)

Fig. 6.1 *(a)* 16 s saturation recover image (TR = 250 ms) illustrating the paradoxical enhancement due to blood flow; *(b)* slight aliasing in the vertical direction caused by cardiac motion; *(c)* effect of random patient movement; *(d)* localised area of zero signal due to the presence of metallic object adjacent to the head; *(e)* the effect of a larger ferromagnetic object in the region of the upper chest; *(f)* image with the Fourier transform artefact

7

Imaging the head and neck

Introduction

The brain was one of the first areas where MRI was applied in the investigation of disease, and is the area where most research has been performed and clinical results obtained. It soon became clear that there were several reasons why MRI would rival CT in the investigation of the brain and in some respects could be superior.

Advantages

MRI has the following advantages

(1) MRI uses non-ionising radiation and appears to be without hazard. The potential hazards which may exist, such as the effects of the magnetic field on pacemakers and aneurysm clips described in Chapter 6, can be avoided as long as the precautions outlined are observed.

(2) The signal intensity of MR images is dependent on three variables (T_1, T_2 and proton density) unlike the single variable in CT (attenuation coefficient). Individual pulse sequences can be altered to highlight any one of the three parameters and thus optimise the investigation to the particular clinical problem. However, this availability of multiple pulse sequences brings with it additional problems in that some types of pathology may be missed if the correct pulse sequence is not used. Also, by employing a multiplicity of sequences the imaging time is inevitably prolonged.

(3) In MRI there are no streaking artefacts which are often found in CT and which can degrade the quality of the image particularly in the posterior fossa.

(4) The availability of direct sagittal and coronal imaging allows very accurate and rapid localisation of intracranial pathology without the relatively high radiation dose and extra time involved in obtaining reformatted information from transverse sections as with CT. Direct coronal and sagittal CT images can now be performed but this is not always possible, perhaps due to technical limitations of the machine, or an uncooperative or unfit patient.

(5) The high contrast levels available in MRI make the use of

contrast agents unnecessary in most instances. However, as we will see later MRI contrast agents may be useful in some cases particularly when one wants to define the border between a lesion and associated oedema.

Normal anatomy

The anatomy displayed on transverse MR sections corresponds closely to that displayed by CT but there are several important differences. There is a very high level of grey-white contrast available, particularly on inversion recovery, and this is greater than even the latest generation of CT scanners can provide. Compact bone gives no signal in MRI, and therefore no signal is seen in the regions of the skull vault, petrous ridges and orbital bones. This phenomenon is useful in two ways: there are no streaking artefacts from bone which can degrade the image in CT and soft tissue structures such as the third, seventh and eighth cranial nerves can be imaged unhampered by surrounding bone. It must be realised that bony manifestations of pathology such as hyperostosis and bony destruction will not be demonstrated.

Sagittal sections. The sagittal plane is particularly useful for demonstrating midline structures. The midbrain, pons, medulla and upper cervical cord are seen in continuity. The optimum sequence for differentiating grey and white matter in the brain stem appears to be a spin echo with a long *TR* and short *TE*. The cerebral aqueduct is demonstrated in over 80% of midline sagittal examinations. The cerebellum and fourth ventricle are clearly seen without the artefacts encountered in CT. The optic chiasm is seen surrounded by CSF in the suprasellar cisterns. The pituitary gland is seen as a region of signal intensity equal to cerebral grey matter immediately below and in front of the optic chiasm. A variable amount of fat in the pituitary fossa gives high signal. Below the gland is the sphenoid sinus which usually contains air and is therefore seen as an area of zero signal. Below and behind the pituitary gland is the clivus. This normally contains fatty marrow and will therefore give a high signal with most sequences because of its short T_1 and long T_2. The clivus is an important landmark and points to the anterior margin of the foramen magnum. The posterior margin of the foramen magnum is identified as an area where the high signal of the occipital diploe stops. The anterior and posterior arches of the first cervical vertebra are seen as circular areas of zero signal, due to cortical bone, surrounding high signal cancellous bone. These three anatomical landmarks: the anterior and posterior margins of the foramen magnum and the first cervical vertebra are very important in assessing the normal anatomical relations in this area, and are particularly important in the assessment of craniovertebral anomalies such as Arnold Chiari malformations.

When taken in conjunction with transverse and sagittal images coronal sections give the third dimension in the three-dimensional assessment of intracranial anatomy. The coronal view is particularly useful in delineating the anatomy of the pituitary region. The bony margins of the pituitary fossa are not demonstrated by MRI, but the important anatomical landmarks which are identified are, laterally, the vascular structures of the cavernous sinus, inferiorly, air in the sphenoid sinus, and superiorly, the optic chiasm. In the orbits the central optic nerve is seen flanked by the bulbar muscles and excellent contrast is provided by the high signal from intraorbital fat. The coronal view allows the confirmation of the intra-axial or extra-axial origin of a lesion to be made and shows the mass effect of space-occupying lesions.

Partial volume effects

There are several areas where the partial volume effects may cause problems in cerebral MRI: (1) grey matter in the cerebral sulci may produce an apparently high T_1 area in the white matter on inversion recovery sequences; (2) in the brain stem partial volume averaging with CSF may cause linear artefacts at the pontomedullary and pontomesencephalic junctions. (3) Partial volume averaging may cause some difficulties in the visualisation of small lesions such as acoustic neuromas where thinner slice sections should be employed if possible.

Pulse sequences

Due to the wide variety of MR imagers and field strengths at present in use it is impossible to specify MRI parameters in a dogmatic manner. In this section emphasis will be placed on the variation of the MR image caused by variations of the three basic MRI variables (T_1, T_2 and proton density) plus the additional effect of flow.

Saturation recovery images

Saturation recovery images will demonstrate variations in proton density but will, like all MRI sequences, have a T_1 dependence and so areas of very long T_1 such as CSF, although having a high proton density, give a low signal. Regions of high proton density will usually give a high MRI signal on saturation recovery sequences. Only small variations in proton density occur in disease, and therefore saturation recovery sequences are relatively insensitive to pathological change. One exception to this is the increased proton density seen in an area of intracerebral haemorrhage. This increase is usually greater than that observed in other mass lesions such as tumours. Saturation recovery sequences do, however, have better spatial resolution than inversion recovery sequences.

Inversion recovery images

The most striking feature of inversion recovery images is the excellent contrast which is achieved between grey and white matter. This contrast is very useful in assessing subtle pathology where the only sign may be the loss of this grey–white interface. This level of contrast is also very useful in assessing progressive myelination in children and the mass effects of space-occupying lesions. One very important feature of inversion recovery images is the relationship between TI and the T_1 of the tissue being imaged. If TI is long (compared to the average T_1) then the net magnetisation in the longitudinal plane will have almost recovered to equilibrium and the observed signal will be large. If however the TI is short then the longitudinal magnetisation will have recovered only a little and the signal will be smaller. There is a value of TI where the signal from a particular T_1 tissue will be zero. Inversion recovery images of this tissue with TI values below this 'critical' value will appear like negatives of those images with TI values above it. In general, regions of long T_1 appear dark on inversion recovery images. Grey matter has a longer T_1 than white matter and thus appears darker than white matter on inversion recovery images and this provides the basis for the excellent contrast observed between these two tissues. T_1 is increased in most types of pathology including neoplasia, ischaemia, demyelination and infection. It must be remembered that not all neoplasms have an elevated T_1. More neoplasms are being recognised which have a relatively short T_1. These include malignant melanomas, tumours into which there has been some haemorrhage and other isolated examples with no obvious explanation for the short T_1. Regions of long T_1 are seen as areas of low signal intensity. These may be confused with areas of low proton density that may be seen in areas of calcification which will also give low signal. Differentiation between these two different tissue types can be made by altering TR and TI causing the region of long T_1 to change in signal intensity relative to high signal fat, while the region of low proton density will remain of low relative signal intensity. This manoeuvre of changing the relative signal from long T_1 areas by altering *TR* and *TI* is also useful when examining pathology adjacent to other areas of low proton density, and therefore low signal intensity, such as occur in the compact bone of the skull vault and petrous bones.

Spin echo

In general, images using the spin echo pulse sequence become noisier on increasing *TE* due to a general decrease in the signal intensity. CSF appears darker than brain on short *TE* sequences and gives increasingly higher signals on increasing *TE*. In general, areas with a short T_2 appear dark and vice versa. There is some T_1 dependence in spin echo with a decreased signal if the T_1 is very long. In short *TR* spin echo sequences there is little contrast seen between grey and white matter with the grey matter appearing as a lower signal compared to white matter. This contrast is increased by lengthening *TR* when the grey matter signal intensity increases. This contrast is increased even further on lengthening *TE*. Most pathology including demyelination, neoplasm and infarction is characterised by a prolonged T_2 relaxation time. These changes are best seen on sequences with long *TR* and long *TE* times which also define normal anatomy well and therefore appear to be the optimum type of spin echo sequence. If T_1 information is required from spin echo sequences they can be made more T_1 dependent by decreasing *TR*. Spin echo sequences also appear to be the optimum type of sequence to outline the oedema associated with pathology but even with long *TR*, long *TE* sequences this definition may be inferior to contrast-enhanced CT, and it is here that the paramagnetic contrast agents may have the most crucial role (Figs. 7.1 to 7.10—normal head and neck images).

Important MRI signs

Short T_1

Seen in acute haemorrhage (days) and clot, and fatty lesions such as lipomas.

Long T_1

Seen in infarction, very recent haemorrhage (hours), chronic haemorrhage, demyelination, abscess, arteriovenous malformation, neoplasm and oedema. Remember, however, the occurrence of short T_1 neoplasms mentioned previously (p. 81).

Very long T_1 (approaching CSF values)

Seen in porencephalic cyst and subdural hygromas.

Long T_2

Most pathology which shows a lengthened T_1 will also display an increase in T_2. It may be that this T_2 change is seen in more types of pathology making spin echo sequences the most sensitive of the MRI sequences in the detection of disease. Fat has a long T_2 as does acute haemorrhage, although the latter may have a relatively normal T_2 time with values approximating to white matter.

Increased proton density

Seen in acute infarction, haemorrhage, oedema and tumour.

Miscellaneous

Sometimes the only changes which may be seen are localised areas of loss of grey–white matter contrast or a more diffuse increase in T_1 and/or T_2 relaxation times throughout the white matter as may occur in multiple sclerosis. Mass effects from space-occupying lesions, such as displacement of the brain stem by acoustic neuromas and distortion of the ventricular system by intrinsic tumours, are often better appreciated by MRI than by CT. This is most often due to the increased tissue contrast of MRI and the multiplanar facility.

Neoplastic disease

MRI is an extremely sensitive technique in the investigation of intracranial neoplasms. Many of the reasons for this have been outlined at the beginning of this chapter but several other points must be stressed. There is a broad spectrum of relaxation times found in neoplastic disease and since the signal intensity and contrast in the MRI image depends at least in part on these times it must always be remembered that not all types of tumour will be shown by a single MRI pulse sequence. Calcification is not imaged directly by MRI but its presence is inferred by areas of zero signal. The presence of calcification may be an important clue to the presence of a neoplasm and the lack of this information may be considered critical. However, the lack of this information may be more than compensated for by the demonstration of MRI signs such as regions where the grey–white contrast is lost or where the relaxation times are seen to be abnormal. The margin between tumour and associated oedema may not be as well shown by MRI than by contrast-enhanced CT. Paramagnetic agents may prove to be crucial here.

Intrinsic tumours

Most cerebral tumours display an increase in both T_1 and T_2 times, and therefore, in general, are seen as areas of low signal on inversion recovery images and high signal on spin echo sequences. As previously discussed several tumours have short relaxation times and these include fatty tumours, haemorrhagic tumours and melanomas. Astrocytomas, acoustic neuromas and metastases generally have longer relaxation times than meningiomas. There is, however, a significant overlap in the relaxation times of these tumours. There is also some overlap in the measured relaxation times between some benign lesions and malignant lesions, and it is therefore impossible to predict a histological type from a measured relaxation time. In summary these relaxation time changes are sensitive parameters but are non-specific in diagnostic terms. However when a 'baseline' relaxation time has been obtained at the initial investigation subsequent measurements of this may be useful in assessing response to therapy. There appears to be an initial increase in relaxation times after radiotherapy, followed by a gradual decrease to a level from which deviations can be observed. The multiplanar facility of MRI is particularly useful in the assessment of intrinsic cerebral tumours. The exact extent of the tumour may be difficult to assess due to the previously mentioned problem of separating tumour from associated oedema, but paramagnetic agents should solve this problem. The sagittal plane provides immediate localisation of midline or brain stem lesions by virtue of observed abnormal signal and contour unhampered by CT artefacts. Parasagittal sections may be useful in defining the position of some tumours such as acoustic neuromas and meningiomas. Coronal images confirm the precise location and relations of pathology and can be particularly useful in the temporal and occipital regions. Coronal sections also help to confirm the intra-axial origin of intrinsic brain stem tumours. The effects of a tumour such as displacement of the ventricular system and hydrocephalus will be shown on coronal as well as transverse images, and when both images are viewed in conjunction a very accurate assessment of any mass effect can be made. Parasagittal and coronal sections can be very useful in determining the extracerebral origin of a meningioma which, because of its locally invasive effects, may mimic an intrinsic tumour. The lack of bony artefact is a major advantage of MRI, and in the investigation of intrinsic tumours this is particularly useful in the assessment of tumours of the posterior fossa, brain stem, temporal lobes and those adjacent to the foramen magnum (Figs 7.11 to 7.29—intrinsic tumours in neoplastic disease).

Extrinsic tumours

The pituitary gland, being a midline structure, is readily investigated by MRI and is easily viewed on midline sagittal sections. The midline sagittal plane readily defines the relations of pituitary pathology and, taken in conjunction with coronal sections, assesses this is relation to the optic chiasm above and the cavernous sinuses with the carotid arteries on either side. Even small degrees of suprasellar extension can be easily demonstrated. The bony margins of the pituitary fossa are not shown. This is a disadvantage since the effects of pathology such as bony destruction of the clinoids and expansion of the sella will not be seen. However, this will be offset in most instances by the direct demonstration of intrasellar and suprasellar lesions.

Another important immediate relation to the pituitary gland is the clivus. This normally contains fat which is easily recognised on MR images by its short T_1, long T_2 and high proton density. This appearance is drastically altered by extension of pathological processes from the pituitary gland which are most often neoplastic. This extension will usually result in a lengthening of the relaxation times. This change, from the normal short T_1 of fat to the long T_1 of disease, will be demonstrated particularly well on T_1 weighted images. There is no correlation between the relaxation times of pituitary tumours and the tumour type, although it can be inferred that haemorrhage has occurred into a tumour if the T_1 is noted to be rather low.

The relatively poor spatial resolution of many MR imagers compared to CT is a disadvantage when looking for pituitary microadenomas. This is one area where high field MRI may be useful but another method of improving the image quality would be to increase the amount of signal averaging performed, albeit with the penalty of increasing the overall scan time. This, however, would not be such a great problem in the investigation of the pituitary, where the examination may only consist of a single MR section in each of the three imaging planes. There is usually little problem in differentiating between the different types of pituitary and parapituitary pathologies, many of which cause similar clinical symptoms. Vascular anomalies such as aneurysms are easily identified and their nature confirmed by flow-dependent sequences. The suprasellar origin of pathology such as craniopharyngiomas and hypothalmic lesions can be further confirmed when, in addition to the more accurate anatomical localisation provided by MRI, the pituitary is seen to be normal. Lack of evidence of calcification is perhaps a drawback, but good quality skull films should provide this information. The empty sella syndrome can be identified by demonstrating extension of CSF in the suprasellar cisterns into the pituitary fossa. The relationship of pituitary pathology to the third ventricle is particularly well seen on coronal sections (Figs. 7.30 to 7.45—lipomas, pituitary and parapituitary tumours, and base of skull and orbit tumours in neoplastic disease).

Acoustic neuromas

This is an area where CT encounters several problems, including streaking artefacts and partial volume averaging. These are remedied by MRI. Intravenous contrast is required with CT in most cases since the lesion is rarely seen without contrast enhancement. Air contrast studies are frequently required for the demonstration of these tumours and even these can have false positives. With MR the normal VIIth and VIIIth nerves can be seen contrasted against the zero signal of the petrous bones. There is sometimes a little fatty marrow in the petrous bones but this is restricted to their medial portions. The same features of displacement of the brain stem and the fourth ventricle which allow identification in CT are readily seen on MRI but with the additional localising features which can be shown by the coronal plane. Care must be taken to choose a pulse sequence with variables which will give a high signal from the tumour but will not result in a high signal from adjacent CSF obscuring the tumour signal. By careful manipulation of the parameters it is possible to see the tumour displacing CSF from the internal auditory meatus.

The greatest advantage of MR over CT in the investigation of these tumours is the ease with which MR can show the intracanalicular component of the tumour, particularly when the tumour is still confined to the intracanalicular compartment. Paramagnetic agents may be of help in defining any associated oedema. In the investigation of acoustic neuromas the sagittal plane is probably the least rewarding of the three available. Also, as in the pituitary, bony detail is not seen and therefore indirect evidence of pathology such as bony erosion is not observed. However, this is not a significant handicap when the additional information available is considered (Figs. 7.46 to 7.53).

Meningioma

This is a tumour which may not be detected by MRI unless particular care is taken. This is due partly to the low contrast which is seen to exist between the tumour and the adjacent brain on most sequences and also to the lack of calcium visualisation. Sequences which emphasise anatomical detail are therefore to be preferred when looking for a meningioma. These are usually of the inversion recovery type where the signal intenisty of the tumour will be of similar intensity to grey matter but lower than white matter. When the lesion has been identified sagittal and coronal sections will allow the dural origin of the lesion to be confirmed. Calcification in a meningioma may sometimes be seen as areas of zero signal intensity.

Demyelinating disease

MR is an extremely sensitive technique in the investigation of white matter disease and demonstrates abnormalities in multiple sclerosis (MS) on a scale comparable to post-mortem findings. With inversion recovery sequences MS lesions are highlighted since the loss of myelin with a short T_1 and the accumulation of fluid with a long T_1 in this type of lesion combine to give areas of markedly elevated T_1 values. Partial volume effects, particularly from the cortical sulci can cause problems in the supraventricular regions. The long T_1 of CSF can also cause problems and create high signal partial volume errors in the periventricular areas. One must therefore be very careful when trying to diagnose MS lesions by inversion recovery techniques. Many of these problems can be overcome by the use of spin echo sequences where, by manipulating the variables, it is possible to keep the signal from CSF low relative to brain and much lower than an MS lesion. Using this type of spin echo sequence there are far fewer problems in the identification of lesions in the supraventricular and periventricular areas. A further advantage of this type of sequence is the reduced contrast achieved between grey and white matter which results in fewer partial volume errors. Another important advantage of MR in MS is the ability to display lesions in the brain stem and cerebellum in patients with negative CT examinations. Lesions in the brain stem and cervical cord are usually shown best by a long *TR*, long *TE* spin echo sequence. Also, by the measurement of relaxation times, it may be possible to monitor the progress of disease.

There are other conditions in which demyelination may be a feature; these include methotrexate encephalopathy, progressive multifocal leucoencephalopathy, carbon monoxide poisoning, Binswanger's disease and most conditions causing cerebral anoxia (Figs. 7.54 to 7.64).

Vascular disorders

Cerebral infarction displays an increase in both T_1 and T_2. Other features of this type of pathology are: (1) Loss of grey/white contrast; on occasions this may be the only recognisable sign. (2) Subtle mass effects which may not be visible on CT. (3) Older infarcts will display other signs analogous to those seen on CT such as widened sulci and compensatory dilatation of the ventricles. These older infarcts often have a central area of longer T_1 values which are close to CSF values. The main advantages of MRI when applied to infarction are better visualisation of cortical involvement due to the lack of bone artefact, and the visualisation of brain stem infarcts due to the multiplanar imaging facility and lack of artefact in the posterior fossa. Unfortunately there are no signs which will make the MR diagnosis of infarction absolute and follow-up scans may be required in a few cases.

Recent haemorrhage is characterised by a short T_1 and long T_2 although very acute haemorrhage appears to have slightly longer T_1 values. A central area of longer T_1 is often seen and in general these relaxation times increase as the haemorrhage becomes more chronic. Areas of calcification can be distinguished from haemorrhage using inversion recovery sequences when the short T_1 haemorrhage will be seen as a high signal while the calcification will be seen as a low signal due to its low proton density. Care must be taken when using inversion recovery sequences to look for haemorrhage as the T_1 of haemorrhage may approximate that of white matter and be missed, although its presence should still be obvious from associated mass effects and oedema.

In haemorrhagic infarction one sees a mixture of the signs of both types of pathology. In subdural haematoma the lesion is easily shown by both inversion recovery and spin echo sequences; generally both T_1 and T_2 are increased but if the bleed is recent the T_1 may be shorter. There is no problem in MR in the recognition of isodense collections and the outer border can be readily seen since there is no bone artefact. Coronal sections are particularly good in estimating the size of the collection. The presence of subarachnoid blood can be established using inversion recovery sequences when its short T_1 allows it to be easily seen in the subarachnoid spaces, contrasted on either side by low signal CSF and low signal bone.

With MR it is possible to identify lesions of cerebral blood vessels such as aneurysms and arteriovenous malformations. However in most instances insufficient information can be obtained regarding feeding and draining vessels and arteriography is still required. Other limitations of MR in the delineation of vascular pathology are its limited spatial resolution and its inability to identify calcification. The main contribution of MR is in the initial demonstration of pathology and it can be very useful in the parasellar region where aneurysms can be located rapidly with parasagittal and coronal sections. The presence of flowing blood within them can be confirmed by flow dependent sequences and thus these lesions can be distinguished from other space-occupying lesions in this location (Figs 7.65 to 7.73).

Infection

Clinical experience with MR in infective conditions is rather limited. Generally, infective processes show increased relaxation times; abscesses may show mass effects but, as with some neoplasms, it may be difficult to separate the associated oedema from the infective focus. The paramagnetic contrast agents may be useful in helping to make this distinction in abscesses as well as in neoplasms. Other infective processes such as the encephalitides can be demonstrated by MR but the changes are non-specific. Since the temporal lobes are shown so much better, due to no bone artefact, the presence of herpes infection which frequently localises to this area should be more easily demonstrated. Infarcts, usually peripheral, are often demonstrated in many forms of meningitis by MRI.

Congenital disorders

Most congenital abnormalities of the brain are well shown by MR. Agenesis of portions of the brain are readily shown but there are no obvious advantages over CT. In *Sturge Weber* syndrome, although the calcification is not demonstrated, there is seen to be loss of grey–white contrast outside the areas of calcification displayed by CT. Abnormalities of midline cerebral structures such as lipoma of the corpus callosum are rapidly assessed, often with dramatic results. The sagittal plane is particularly useful in the assessment of the craniovertebral junction and can be used to display tonsillar herniation in the *Arnold Chiari* malformation, syringomyelia and tumours in the region of the foramen magnum. Other positional abnormalities, such as the relations of the cord to the first cervical vertebra in rheumatoid arthritis and the deformity of the brain stem in basilar invagination, are also well demonstrated (Figs. 7.74 to 7.78).

Miscellaneous

The degree of cerebral and cerebellar atrophy is well shown by MRI;

in particular the cerebellar changes are seen due to the superior demonstration of the posterior fossa by MRI. This may be in isolation or as part of a clinical syndrome such as dementia or alcoholic brain damage. It may be possible to characterise different types of dementia by T_1 measurements of white matter, and also to assess the response to rehabilitation in alcoholics by T_1 analysis. In *Huntington's chorea* MR can assess the volume of the atrophied caudate nucleus very accurately, and relaxation time measurements may be of some predictive value in family members at risk. In *Paget's* disease of bone it is possible to assess the soft tissue component of this disease within the bones of the skull vault.

In trauma cases the previously noted features of haemorrhage and extracerebral collections may be seen. In addition, it should be possible to demonstrate white matter shearing injuries and again the loss of grey–white contrast may indicate damage even when a CT scan appears normal. More examples of trauma cases are required before dogmatic statements can be made regarding evolution of cerebral damage and the difficulties of imaging acute head trauma must be considered. In particular, the amount of ancillary metallic equipment often attached to, or in the vicinity of, the acutely traumatised patient must be considered as must the fact that this type of patient may be uncooperative or require close observation.

In *Wilson's* disease the deposition of paramagnetic copper causes tissue damage leading to an increase of the relaxation times in the thalamus and lenticular areas (Fig. 7.79 to 7.82).

Paramagnetic agents

A paramagnetic agent is a substance which will change the relaxation times of the tissues into which it is introduced. The substance which has the most promise for clinical use in the future is gadolinium. This is normally toxic but, when chelated to DTPA appears to be very safe. Gadolinium DTPA has the effect of reducing the relaxation times of the tissues in which it accumulates and is excreted almost entirely by the kidneys after an intravenous injection. Clinical experience with this compound is still very limited but its main role may lie in its ability to separate tumour from surrounding oedema in the brain. More work is required to determine the optimum pulse sequences and dosage to be used with gadolinium but it appears that sequences of the inversion recovery type with 'medium' values of *TR* and *TI* will probably turn out to be best. Another benefit of paramagnetic agents is that they will allow visualisation of lesions using sequences with a shorter *TR*. This will therefore decrease examination time and increase patient throughput. The use of paramagnetics may also make the detection of 'difficult' lesions, such as meningiomas, more easy.

Paediatrics

There are certain features of MRI which are of particular importance in paediatric imaging.

(1) The lack of non ionising radiation is particularly attractive in the young especially when follow up examinations are being considered.

(2) The superior visualisation of the brain stem and posterior fossa is important since most brain stem gliomas occur in a younger age group and may be difficult to detect by other methods.

(3) A particularly important paediatric application is the ability of MR to clearly demonstrate progressive myelination or any retardation in this process which may occur as a result of such things as birth injury.

(4) The ability of MRI to demonstrate abnormalities in bone marrow has many applications in paediatric practice and may be used to demonstrate the intramedullary spread of primary and secondary tumours, infection, leukaemia and also aplastic anaemia where fatty replacement of the marrow spaces causes an increased fat signal.

(5) The fact that contrast medium and an intravenous injection is seldom required makes the use of MRI particularly attractive for all paediatric patients.

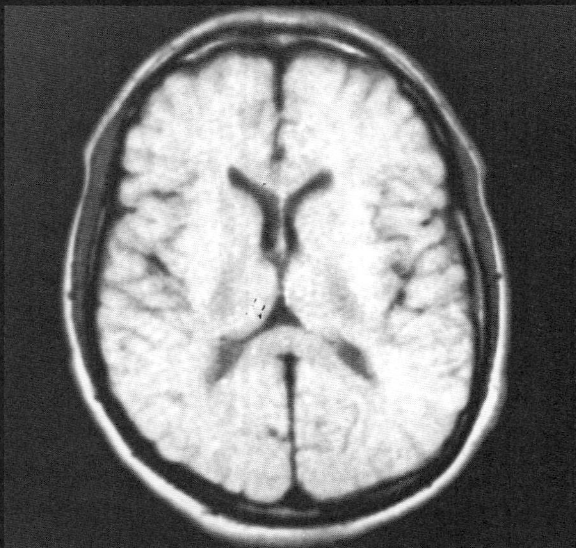

Fig. 7.1 Transverse through ventricles; saturation recovery (courtesy of Hammersmith Hospital)

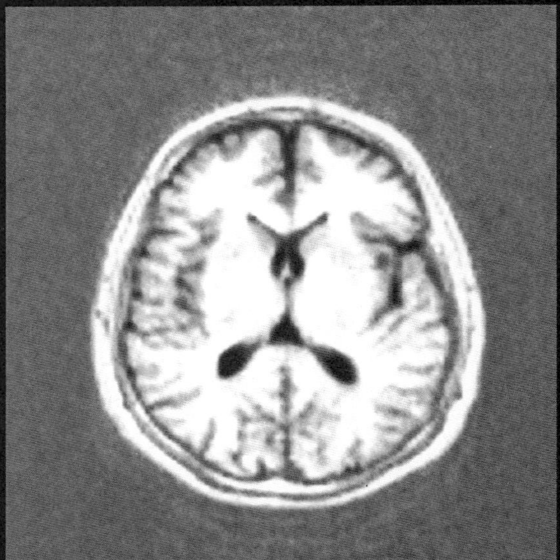

Fig. 7.2 Transverse through ventricles; inversion recovery; (long *TR*)

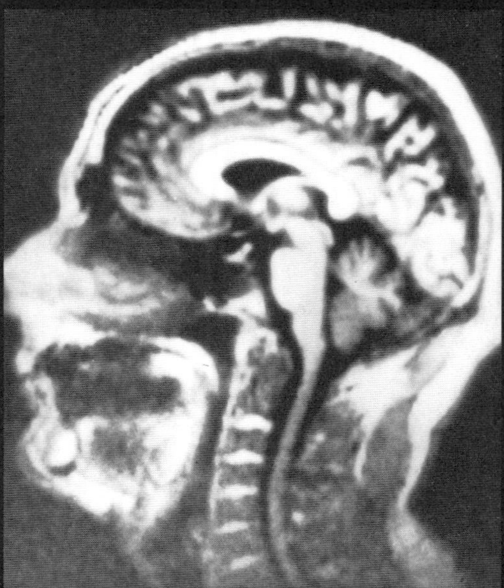

Fig. 7.3 Midline sagittal; inversion recovery; (long *TR*) (courtesy of Hammersmith Hospital)

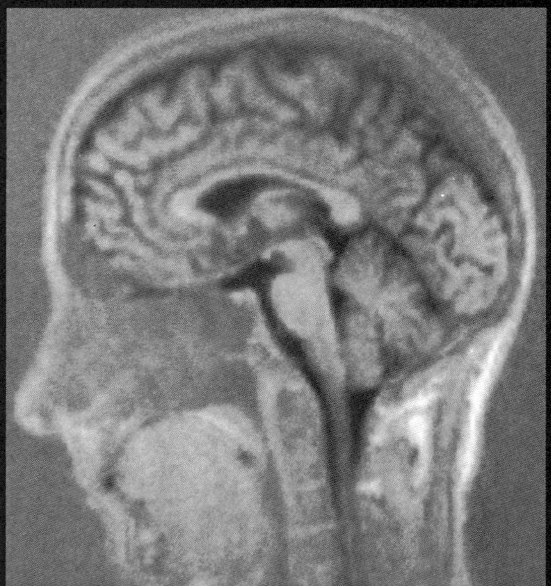

Fig. 7.4 Midline sagittal; inversion recovery

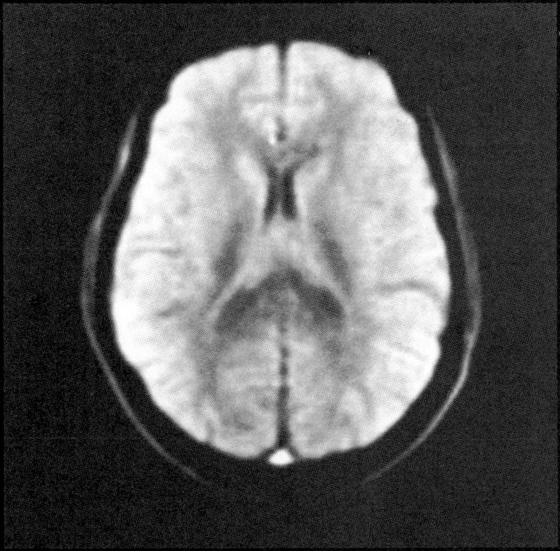

Fig. 7.5 Transverse through ventricles; saturation recovery (courtesy Hammersmith Hospital)

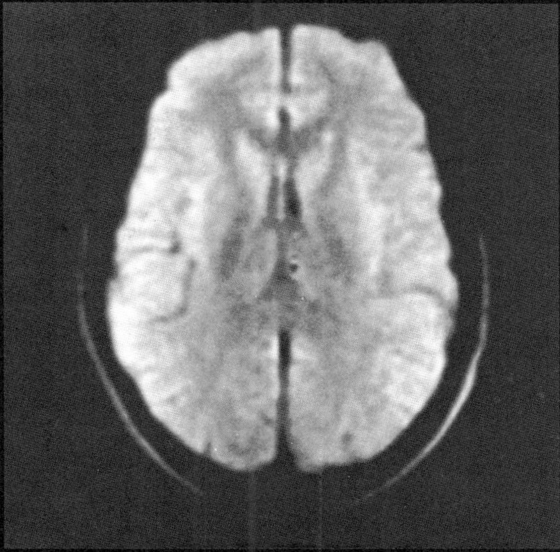

Fig. 7.6 Transverse through ventricles; spin echo *TE* 80 ms (courtesy Hammersmith Hospital)

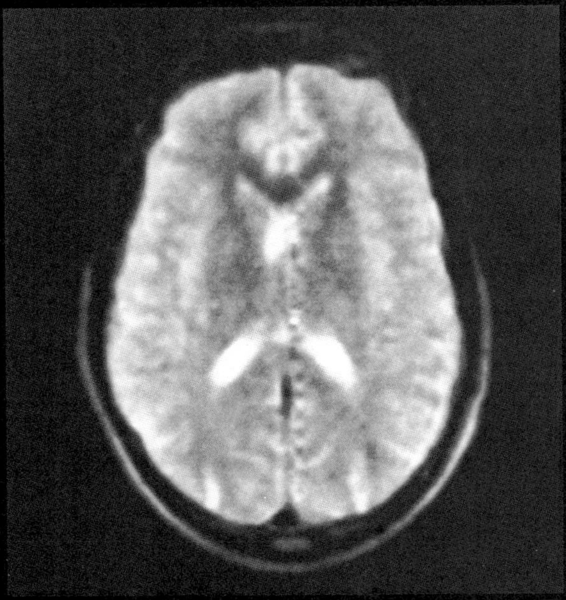

Fig. 7.7 Transverse through venticles; spin echo *TE* 160 ms (courtesy Hammersmith Hospital)

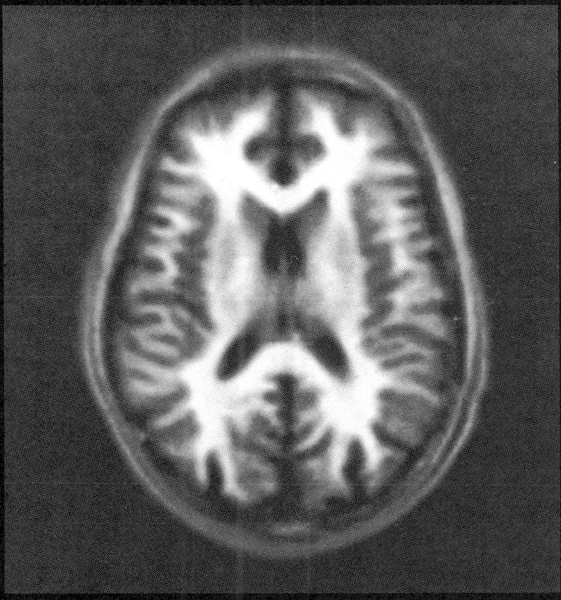

Fig. 7.8 Transverse through ventricles; inversion recovery *TR* 1400, *TI* 400 ms (courtesy Hammersmith Hospital)

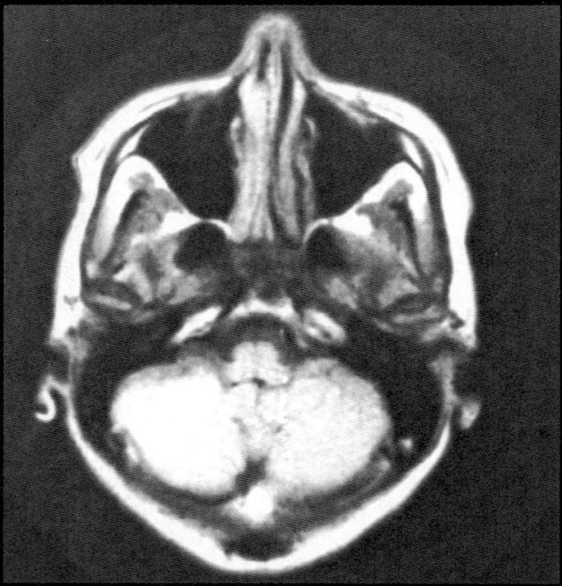

Fig. 7.9 Transverse posterior fossa; spin echo (courtesy Hammersmith Hospital)

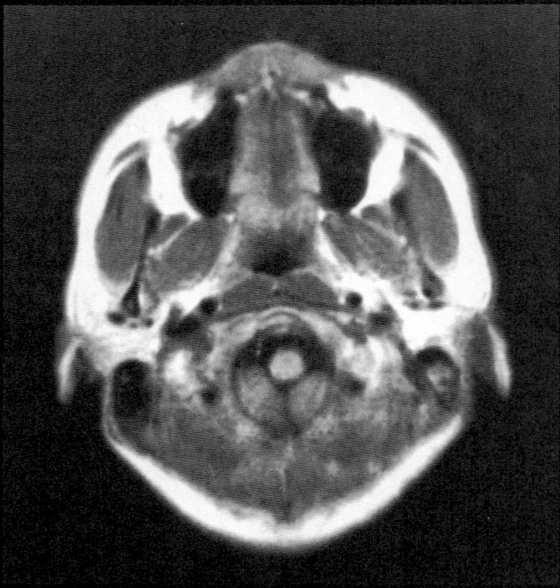

Fig. 7.10 Transverse base of skull; spin echo; (courtesy Hammersmith Hospital)

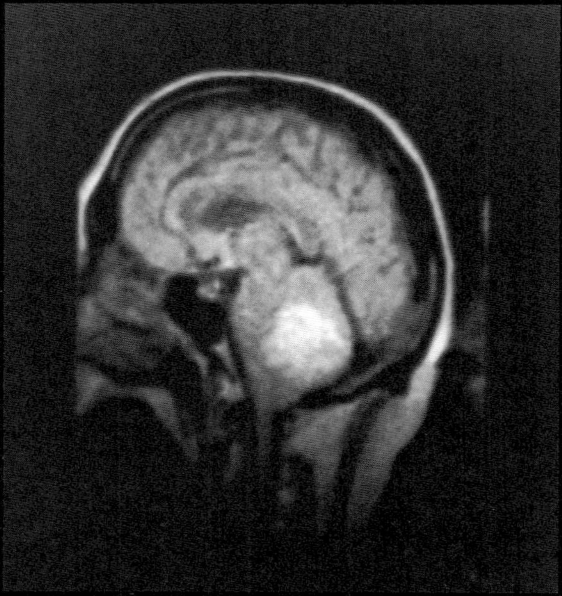

Fig. 7.11 Posterior fossa tumour; spin echo: sagittal (courtesy Hammersmith Hospital)

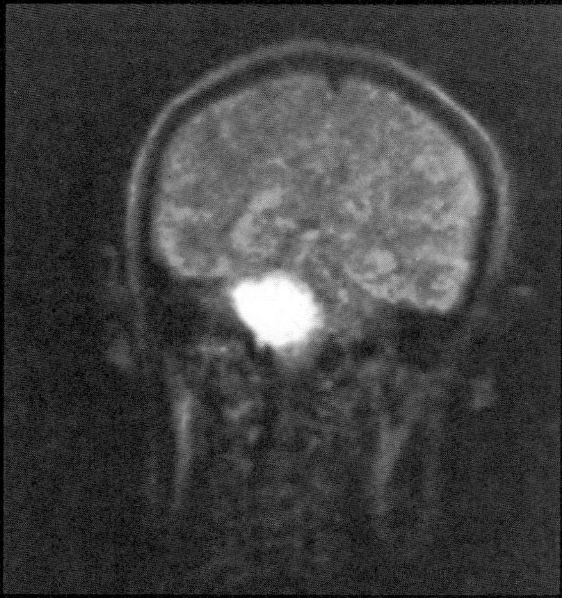

Fig. 7.12 Posterior fossa tumour; spin echo; coronal (courtesy Hammersmith Hospital)

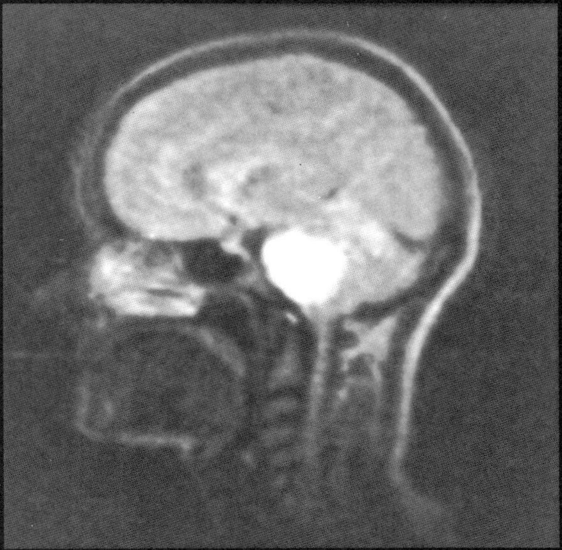

Fig. 7.13 Brain stem tumour; spin echo; sagittal (courtesy Hammersmith Hospital)

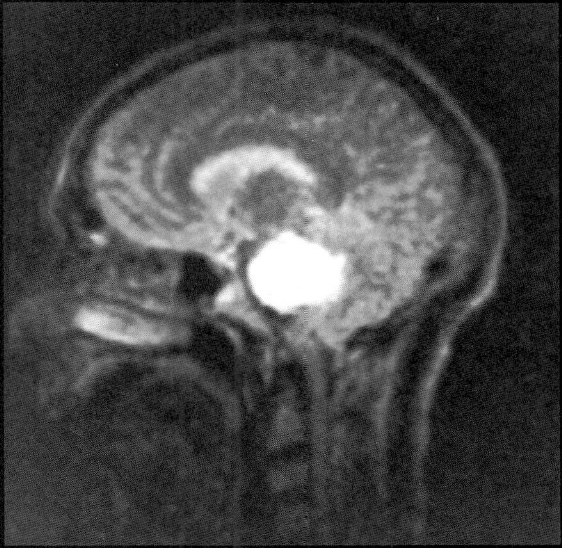

Fig. 7.14 Brain stem tumour; spin echo; sagittal (courtesy Hammersmith Hospital)

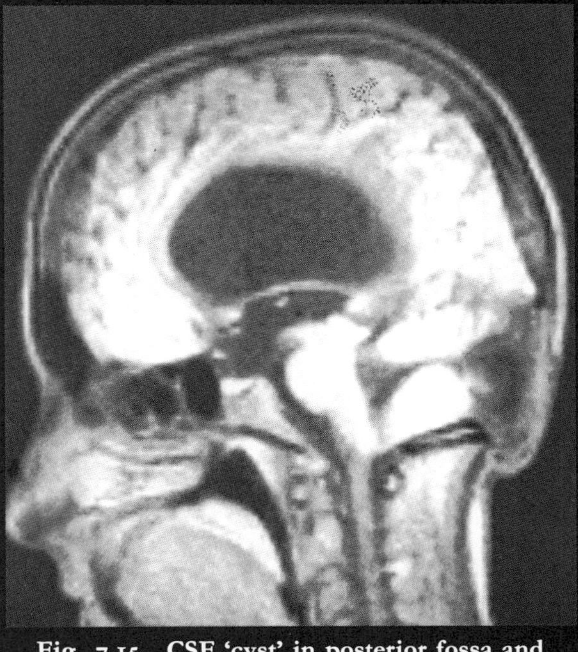

Fig. 7.15 CSF 'cyst' in posterior fossa and hydrocephalus; sagittal; proton density

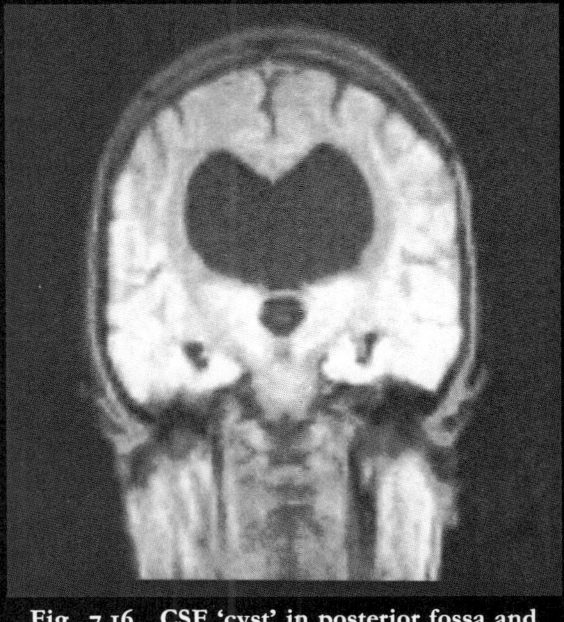

Fig. 7.16 CSF 'cyst' in posterior fossa and hydrocephalus; coronal; proton density

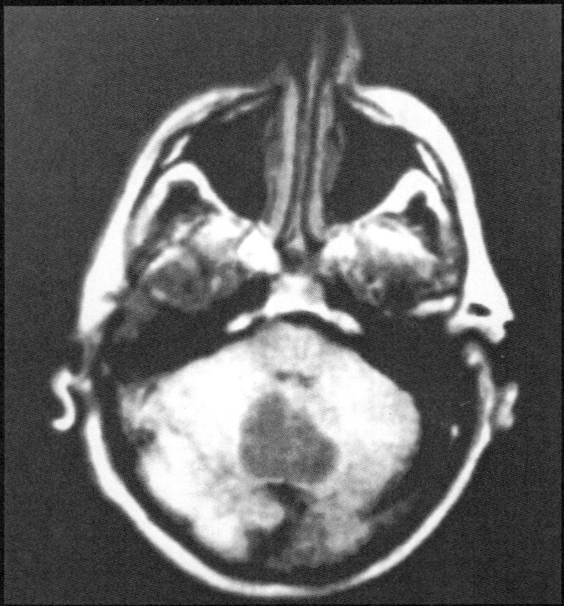

Fig. 7.17 Posterior fossa tumour; inversion recovery; transverse; before gadolinium DTPA (courtesy Hammersmith Hospital)

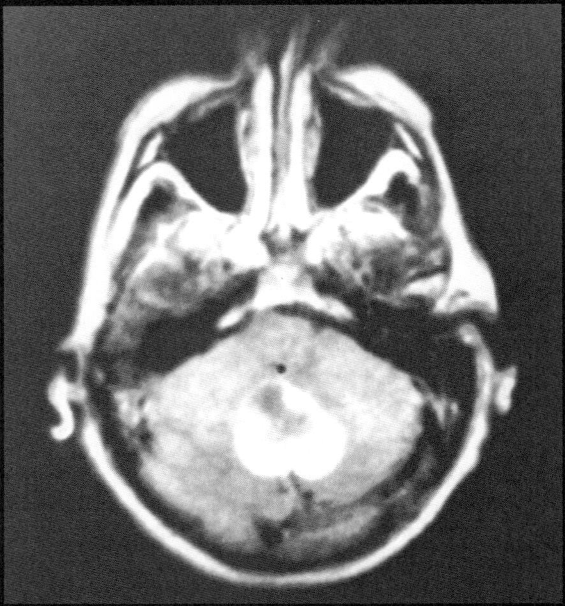

Fig. 7.18 Posterior fossa tumour; inversion recovery; transverse; after gadolinium DTPA (courtesy Hammersmith Hospital)

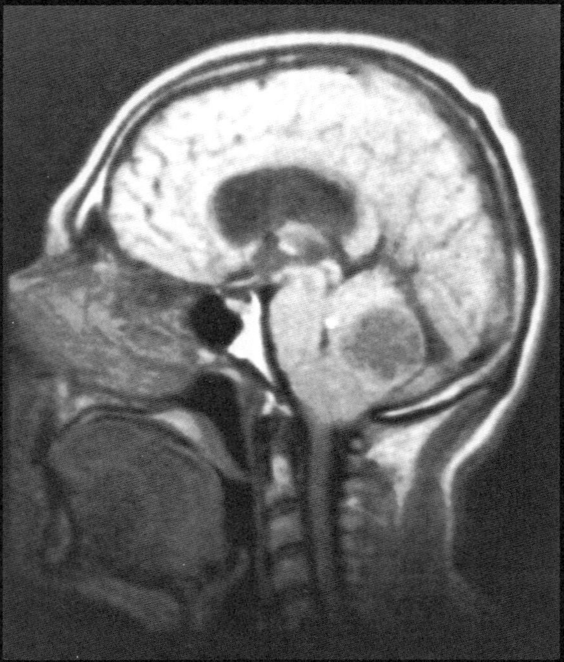

Fig. 7.19 Posterior fossa tumour; inversion recovery; sagittal; before gadolinium DTPA (courtesy Hammersmith Hospital)

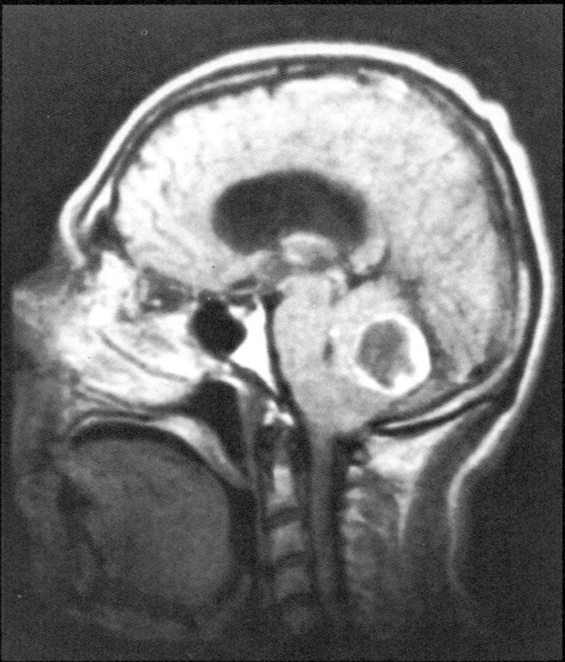

Fig. 7.20 Posterior fossa tumour; inversion recovery; sagittal; after gadolinium DTPA (courtesy Hammersmith Hospital)

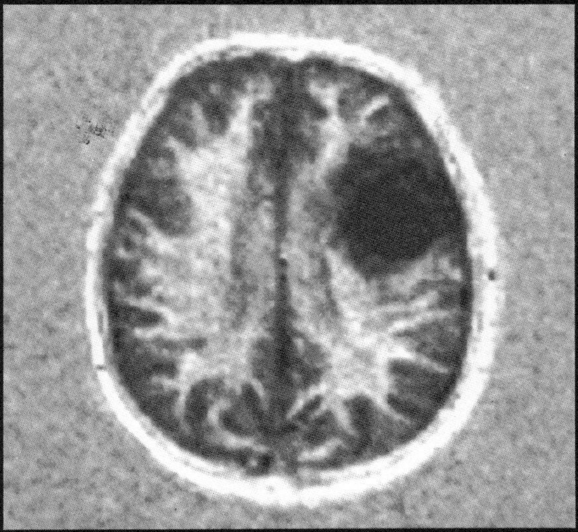

Fig. 7.21 Glioma; transverse, inversion recovery.

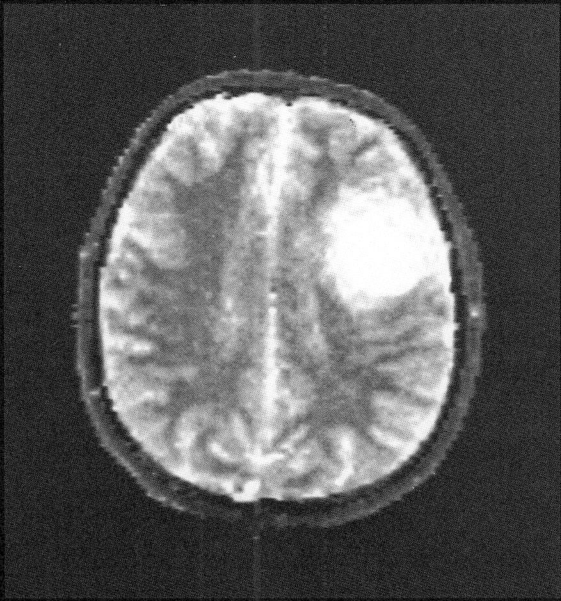

Fig. 7.22 Glioma; transverse; calculated T_1

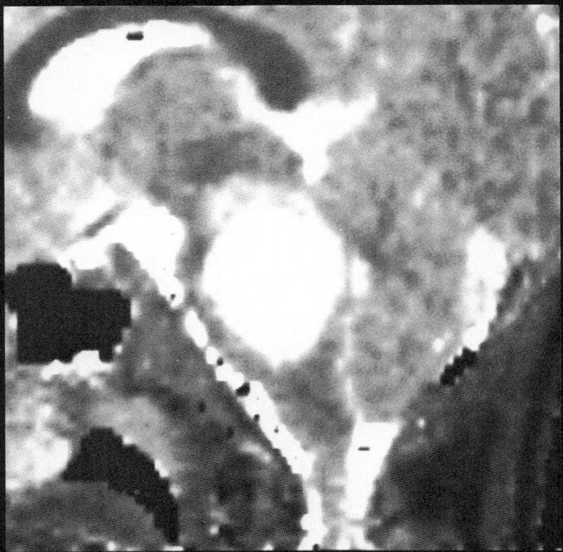

Fig. 7.23 Brain stem glioma; calculated T_1; sagittal

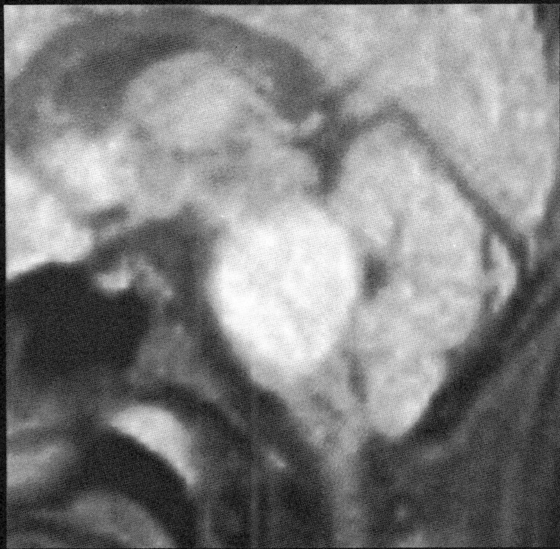

Fig. 7.24 Brain stem glioma; T_1 weighted

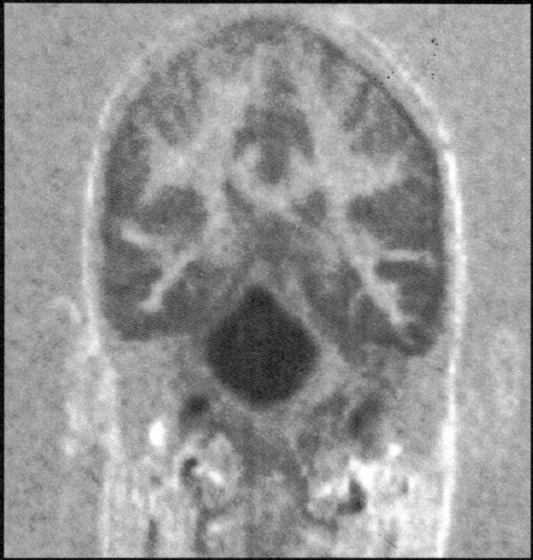

Fig. 7.25 Brain stem glioma; inversion recovery, coronal

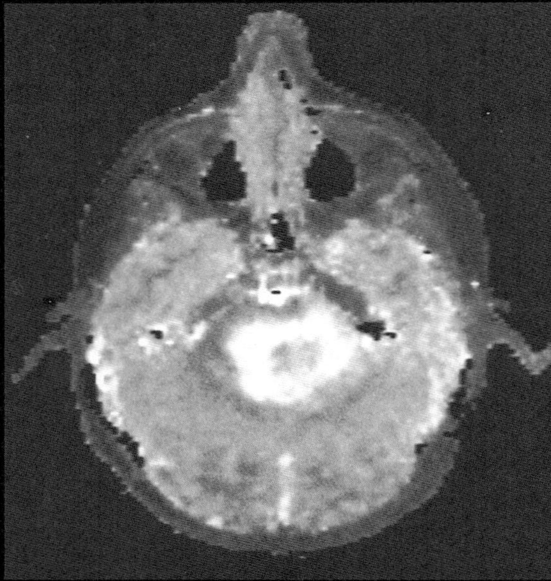

Fig. 7.26 Brain stem glioma with haemorrhage; calculated T_1; coronal

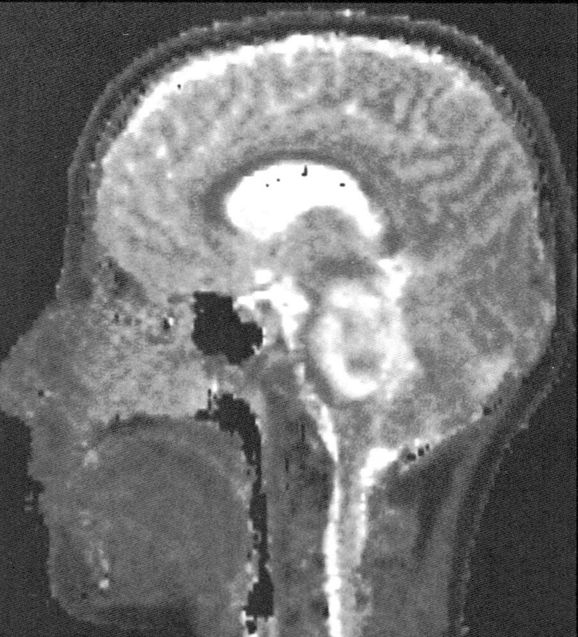

Fig. 7.27 Brain stem glioma with haemorrhage; calculated T_1; sagittal

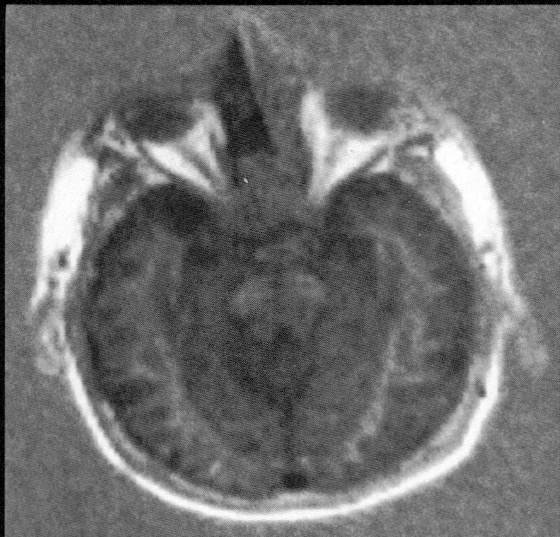

Fig. 7.28 Malignant melanoma deposits; inversion recovery; transverse

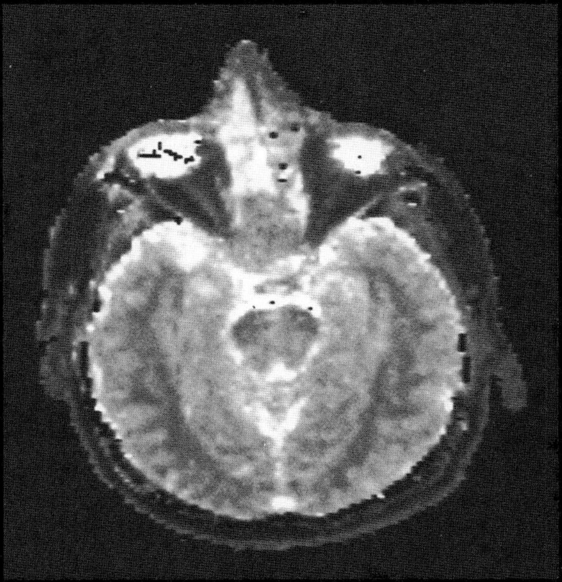

Fig. 7.29 Malignant melanoma; calculated T_1; transverse

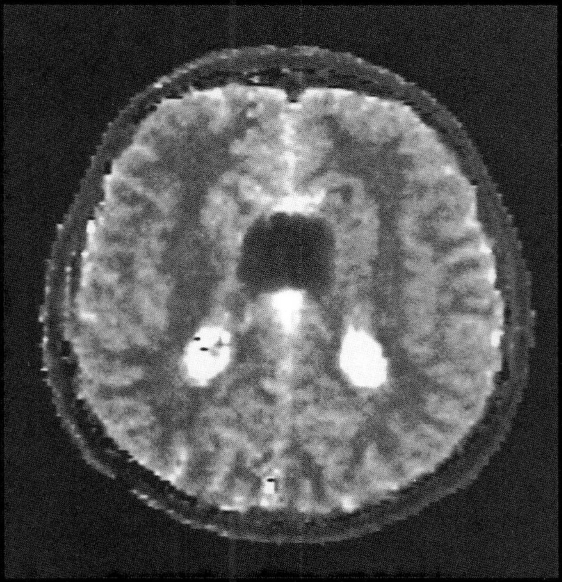

Fig. 7.30 Lipoma with agenesis of corpus callosum; calculated T_1; transverse

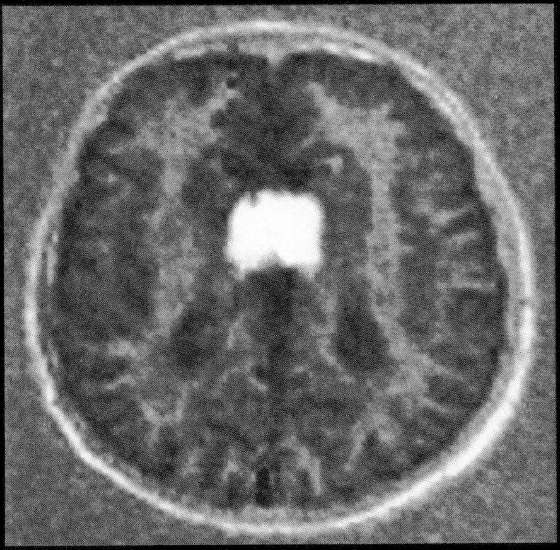

Fig. 7.31 Lipoma with agenesis of corpus callosum; calculated T_1; inversion recovery

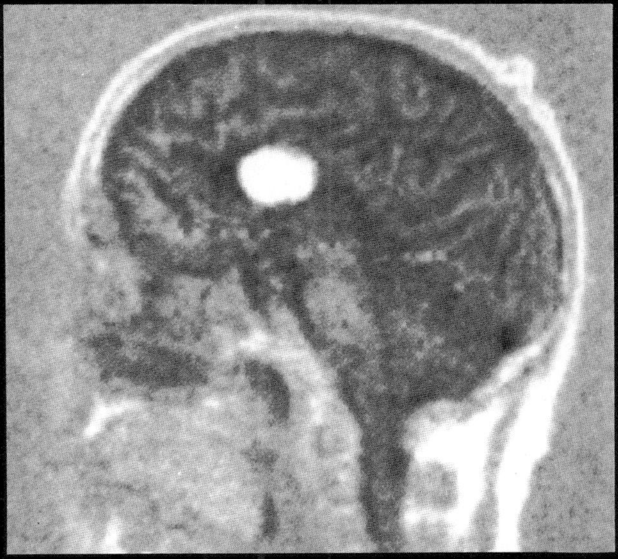

Fig. 7.32 Lipoma with agenesis of corpus callosum; calculated T_1; sagittal

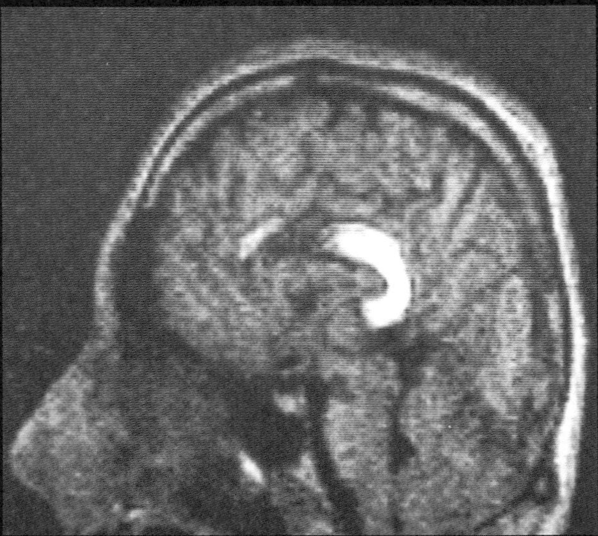

Fig. 7.33 Another example of a lipoma of the corpus callosum; inversion recovery; sagittal

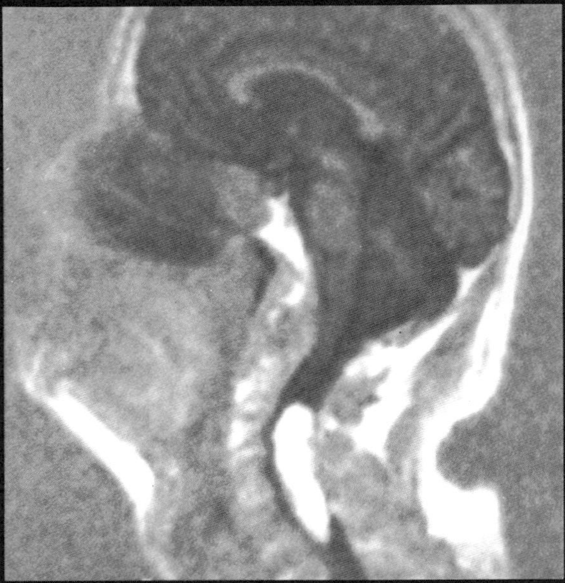

Fig. 7.34 Lipoma of the cervical spinal cord; inversion recovery; sagittal

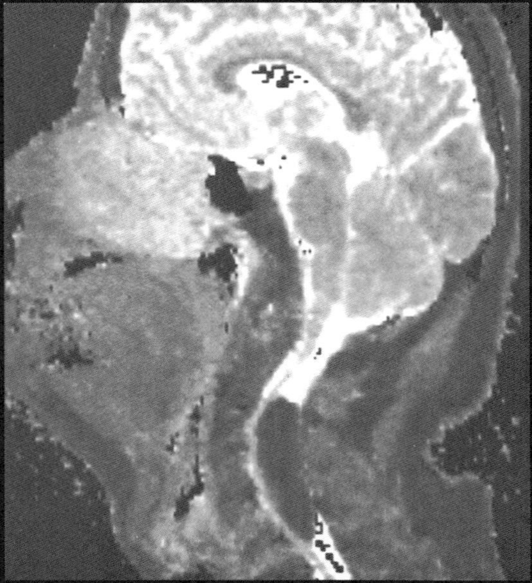

Fig. 7.35 Lipoma of the cervical spinal cord; inversion recovery; calculated T_1

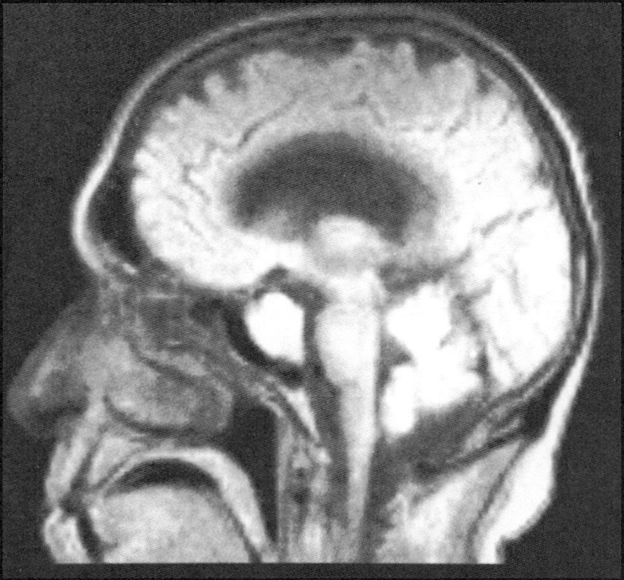

Fig. 7.36 Pituitary macroadenoma; proton density; sagittal

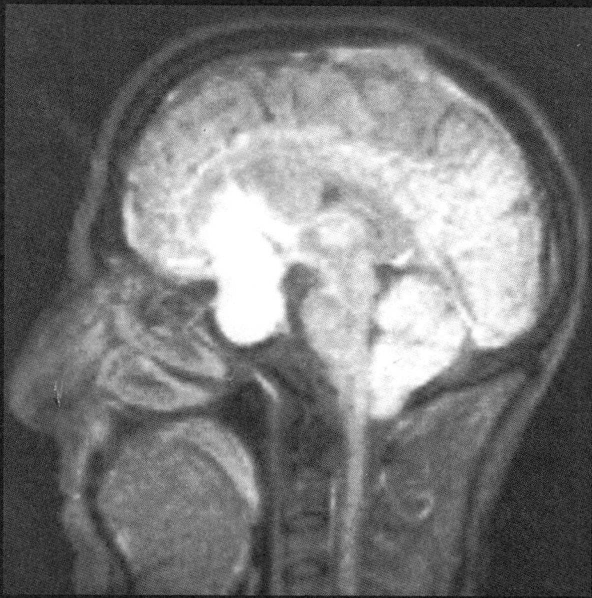

Fig. 7.37 Pituitary macro-adenoma; proton density; sagittal

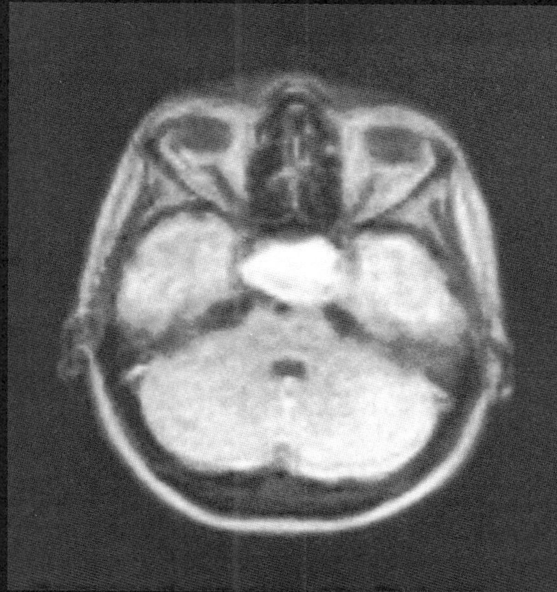

Fig. 7.38 Prolactinoma; proton density; transverse

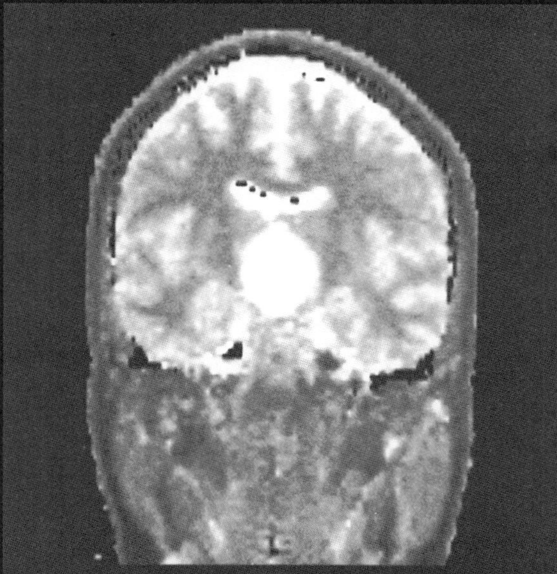

Fig. 7.39 Craniopharyngioma; calculated T_1; coronal

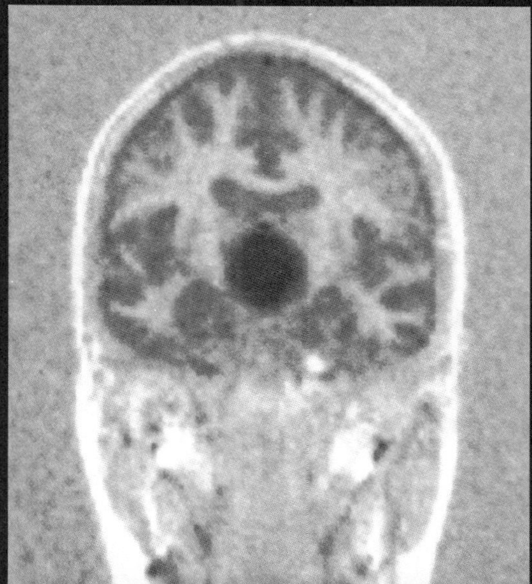

Fig. 7.40 Craniopharyngioma; inversion recovery; coronal

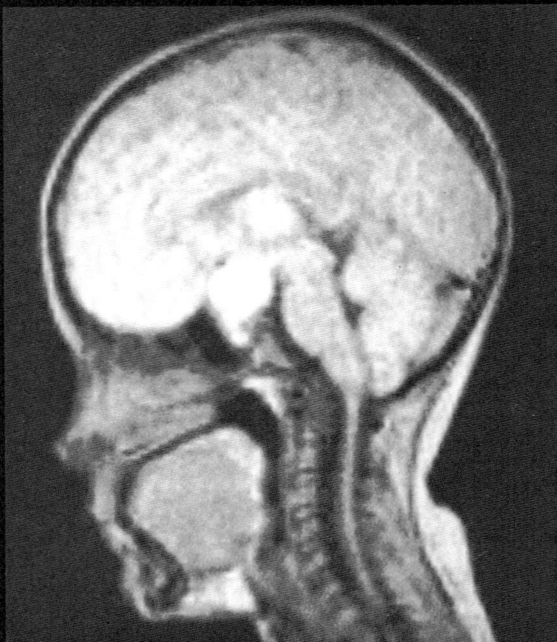

Fig. 7.41 Craniopharyngioma in a child; T_1 weighted image; sagittal

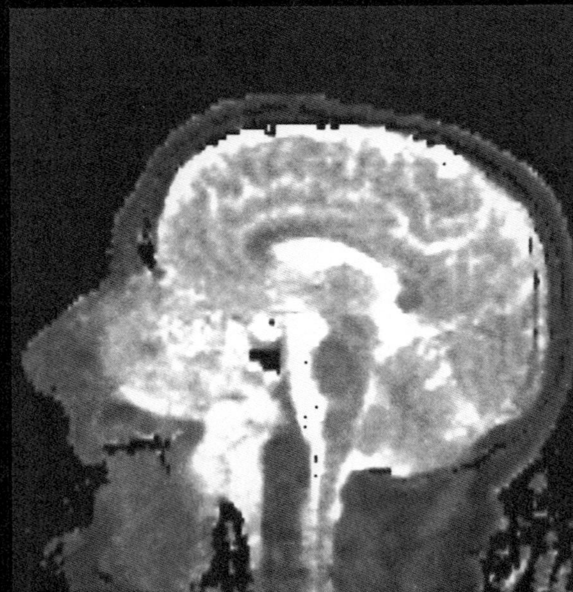

Fig. 7.42 Chordoma, calculated T_1; sagittal

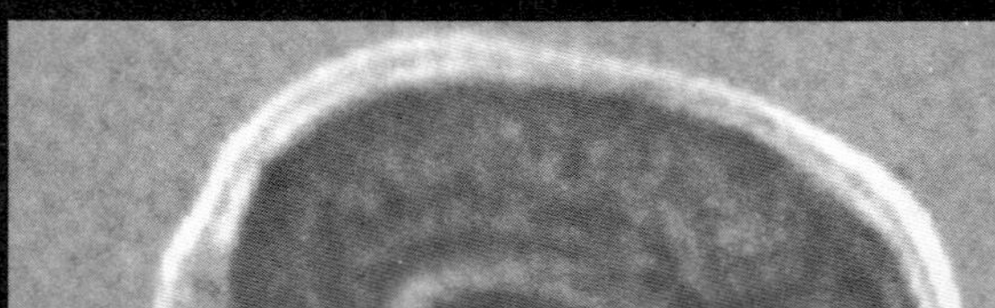

Fig. 7.43 Chordoma; inversion recovery; sagittal

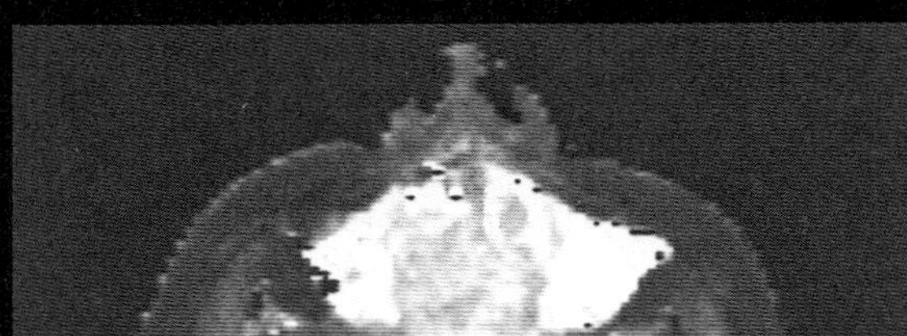

Fig. 7.44 Chordoma; calculated T_1; transverse

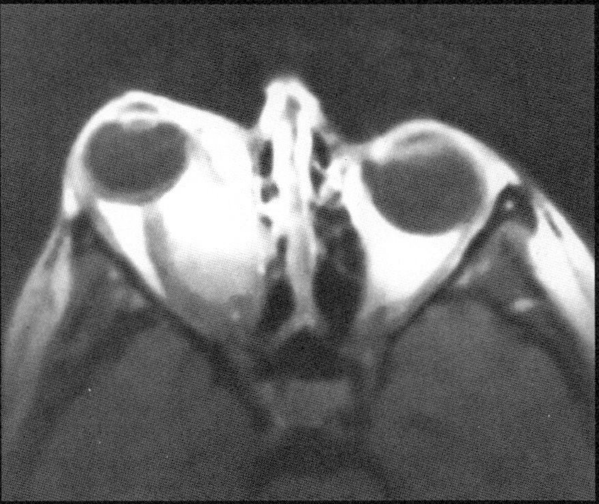

Fig. 7.45 Orbital mass lesion (courtesy Hammersmith Hospital)

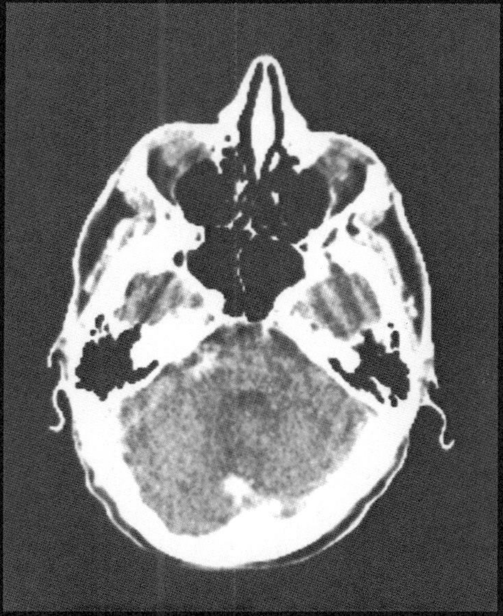

Fig. 7.46 CT acoustic neuroma (courtesy Hammersmith Hospital)

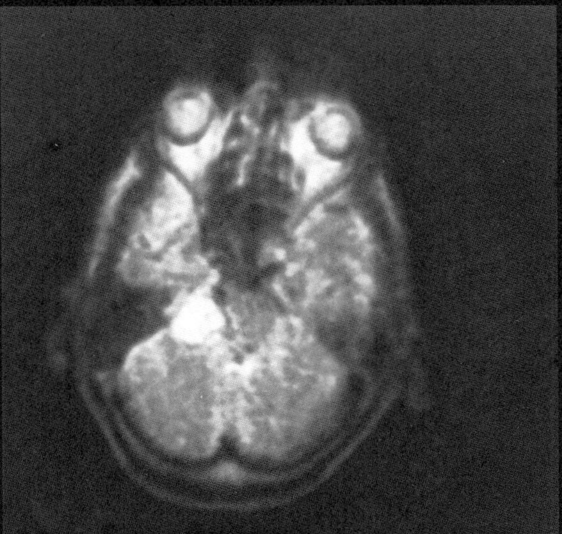

Fig. 7.47 Acoustic neuroma; spin echo; transverse (same example as Fig. 7.46) (courtesy Hammersmith Hospital)

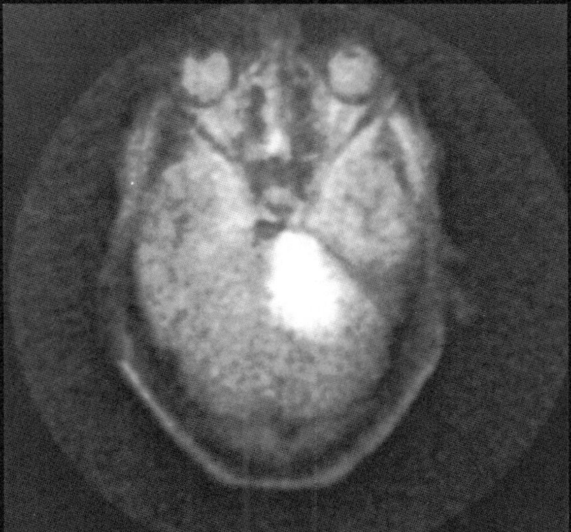

Fig. 7.48 Acoustic neuroma; spin echo; transverse (courtesy Hammersmith Hospital)

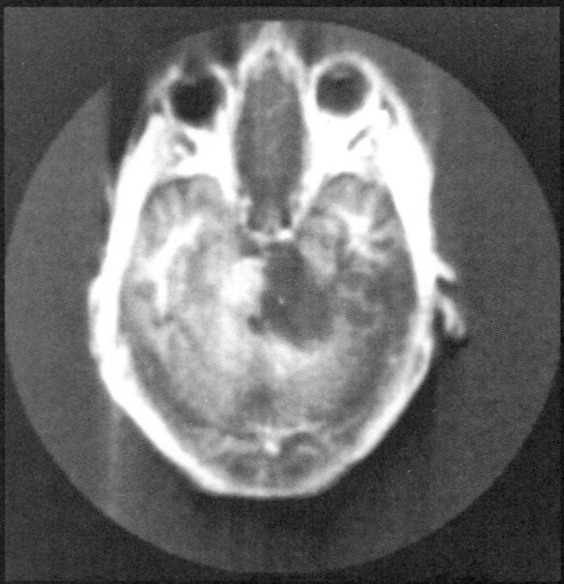

Fig. 7.49 Acoustic neuroma; inversion recovery; transverse (courtesy Hammersmith Hospital)

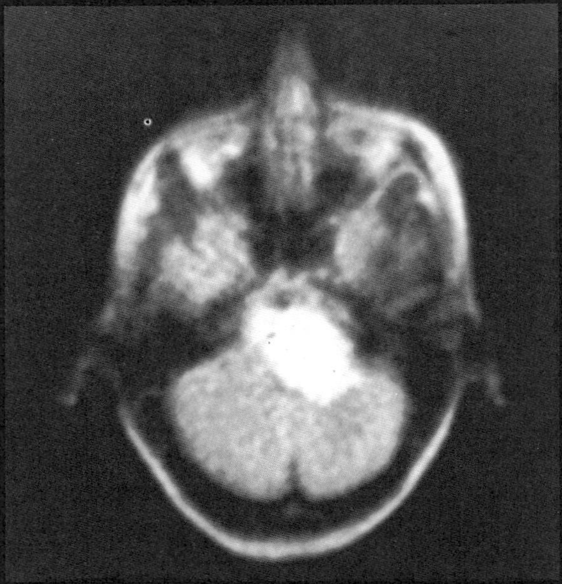

Fig. 7.50 Acoustic neuroma; spin echo; transverse (courtesy Hammersmith Hospital)

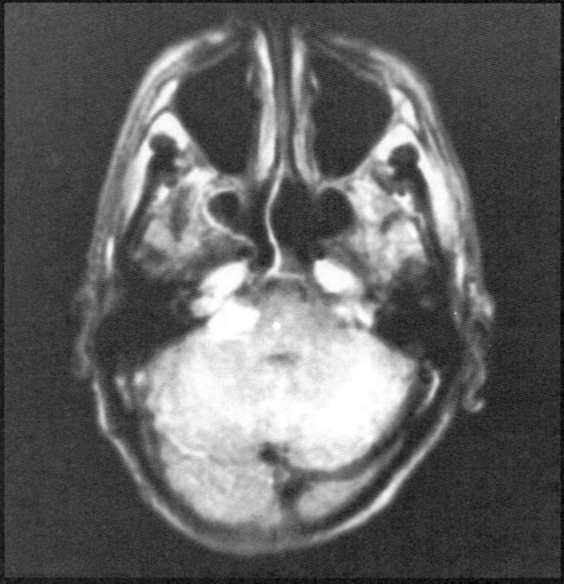

Fig. 7.51 Bilateral acoustics; spin echo; transverse (courtesy Hammersmith Hospital)

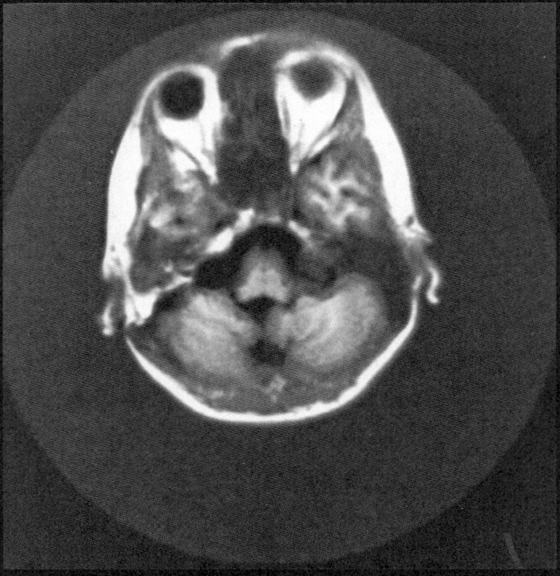

Fig. 7.52 Acoustic neuroma; inversion recovery; transverse; before gadolinium (courtesy Hammersmith Hospital)

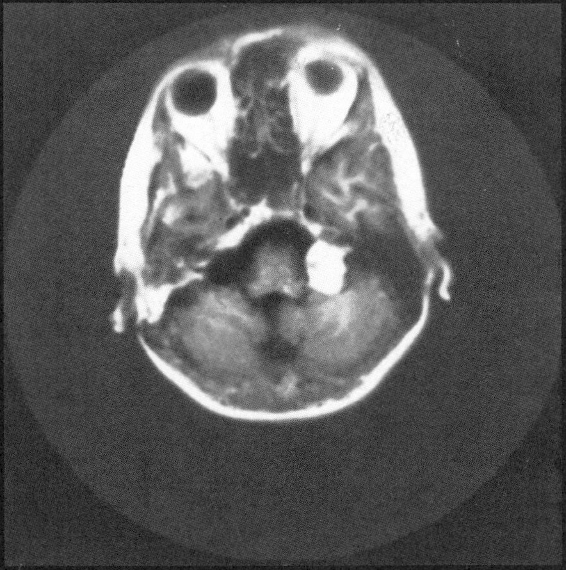

Fig. 7.53 Acoustic neuroma; inversion recovery; transverse; after gadolinium (courtesy Hammersmith Hospital)

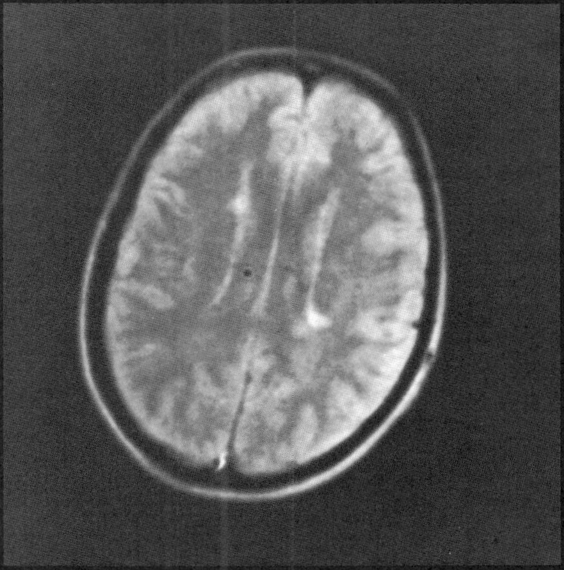

Fig. 7.54 Periventricular demyelination; spin echo; transverse (courtesy Hammersmith Hospital)

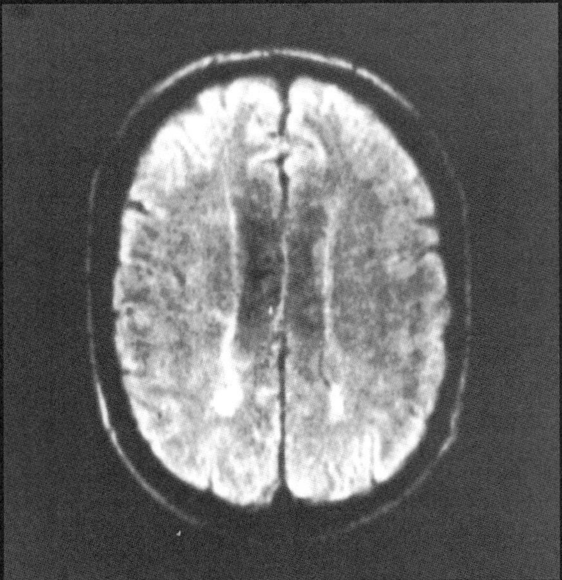

Fig. 7.55 Demyelination; spin echo; transverse (courtesy Hammersmith Hospital)

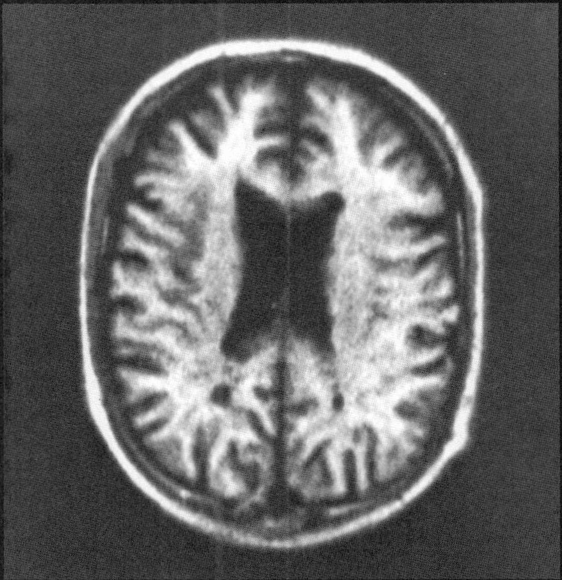

Fig. 7.56 Demyelination; inversion recovery; transverse (courtesy Hammersmith Hospital)

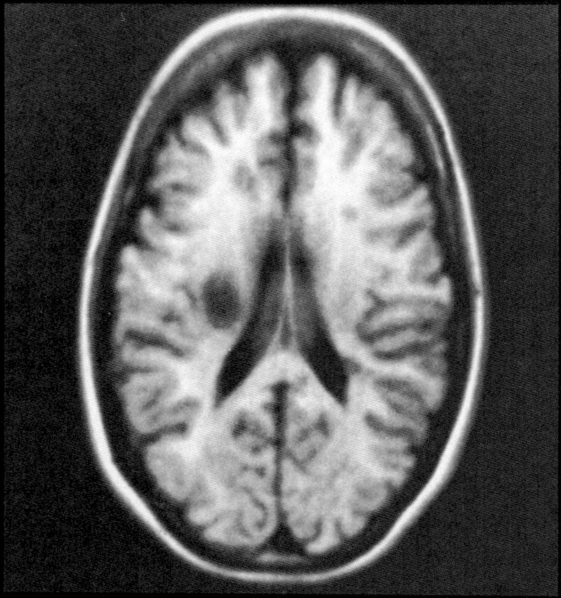

Fig. 7.57 Demyelination; inversion recovery; transverse (courtesy Hammersmith Hospital)

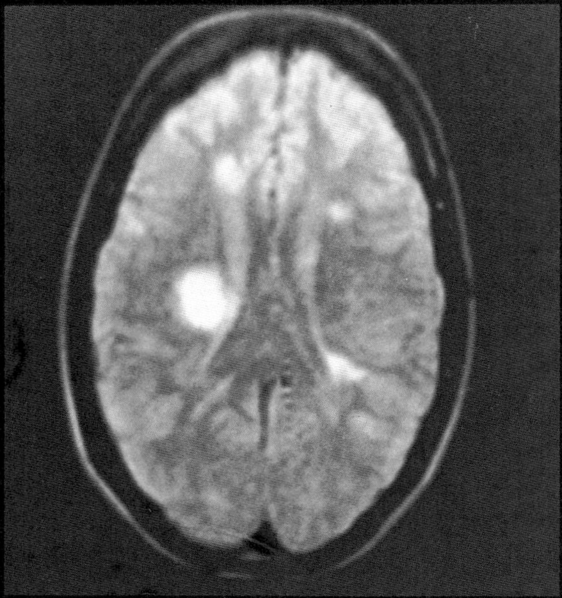

Fig. 7.58 Demyelination; spin echo; transverse (courtesy Hammersmith Hospital)

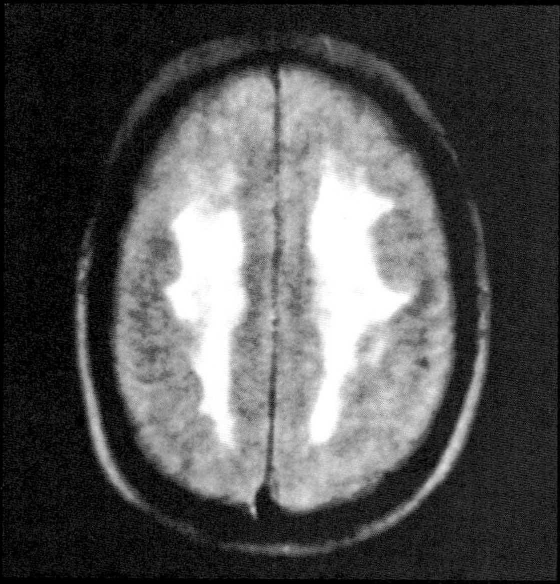

Fig. 7.59 *Binswanger's disease;* spin echo; transverse (courtesy Hammersmith Hospital)

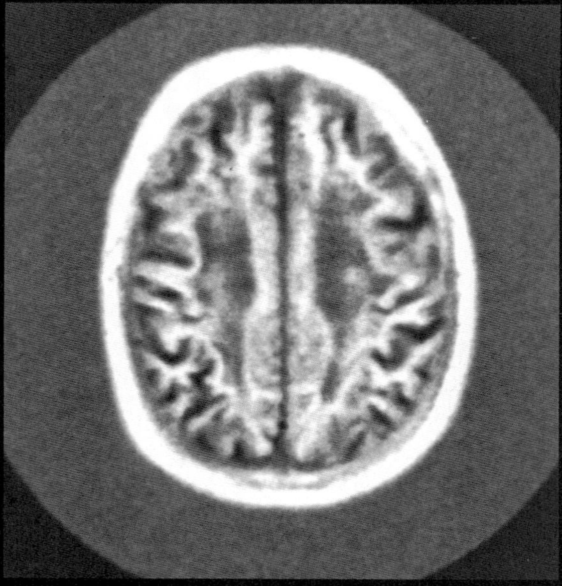

Fig. 7.60 *Binswanger's disease;* inversion recovery; transverse (courtesy Hammersmith Hospital)

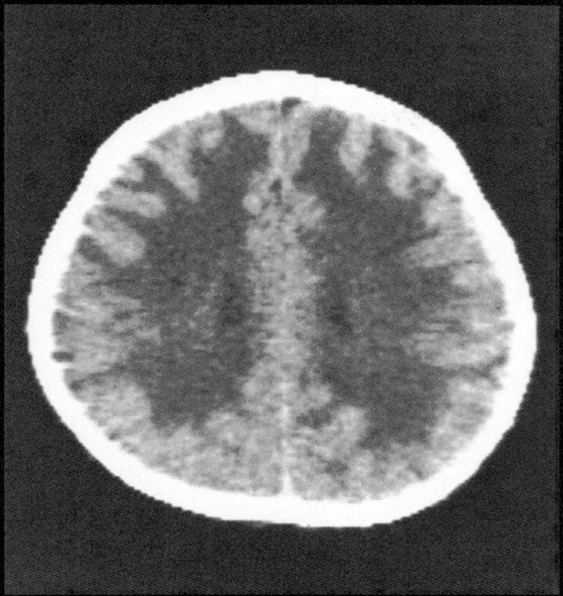

Fig. 7.61 CT Leucodystrophy (courtesy Hammersmith Hospital)

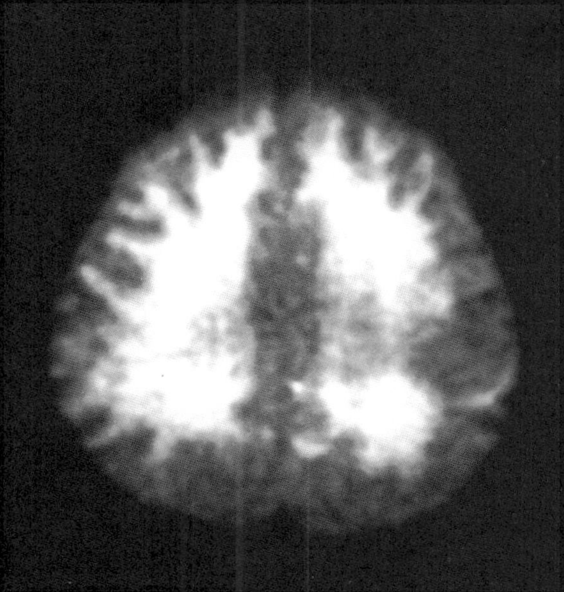

Fig. 7.62 Leucodystrophy; spin echo; transverse (courtesy Hammersmith Hospital)

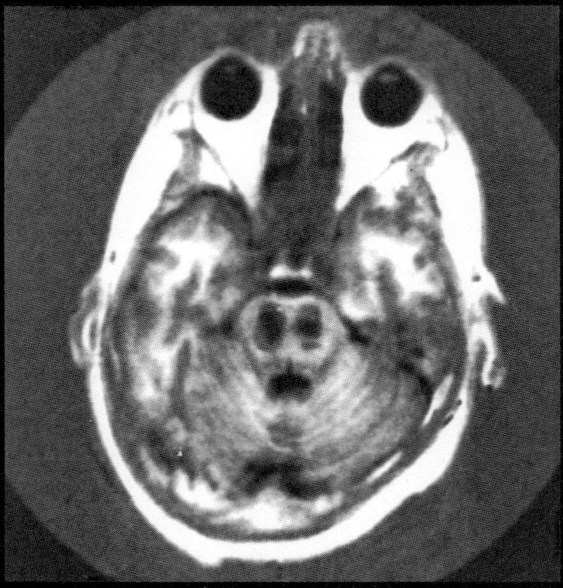

Fig. 7.63 Central pontine myelinolysis; inversion recovery; transverse (courtesy Hammersmith Hospital)

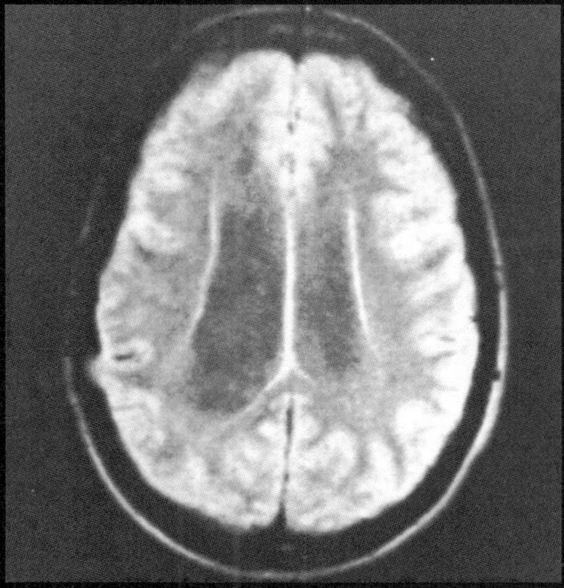

Fig. 7.64 Periventricular high signal; spin echo; transverse (courtesy Hammersmith Hospital)

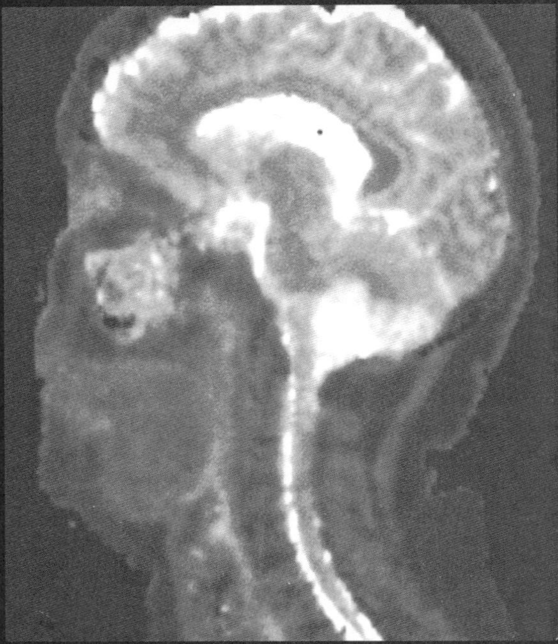

Fig. 7.65 Cerebellar infarct; calculated T_1; sagittal

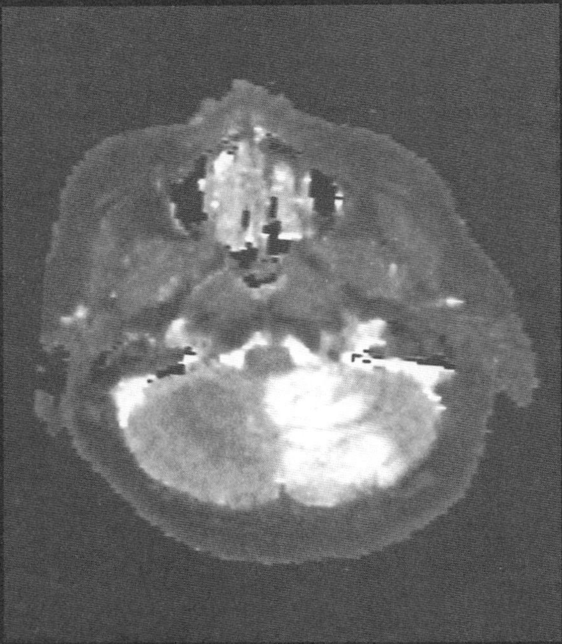

Fig. 7.66 Cerebellar infarct; calculated T_1; transverse

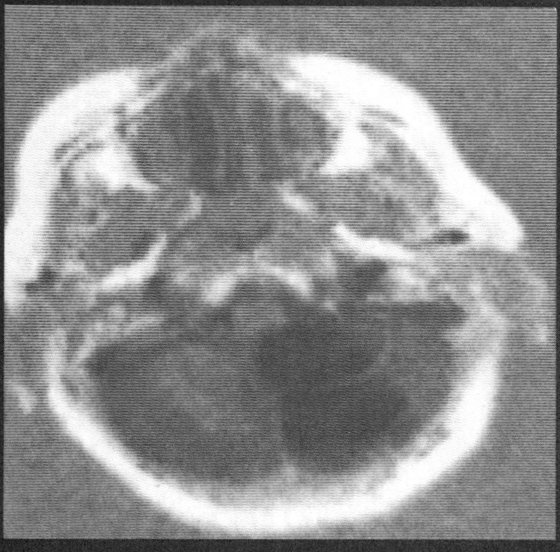

Fig. 7.67 Cerebellar infarct; calculated T_1; inversion recovery

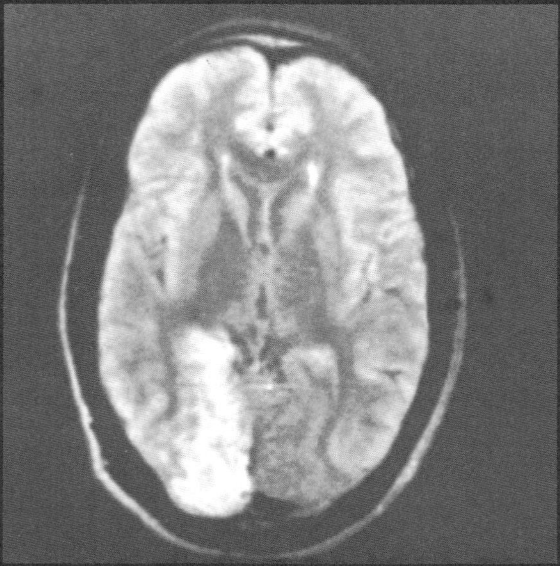

Fig. 7.68 Arteriovenous malformation; spin echo; transverse with gadolinium (courtesy Hammersmith Hospital)

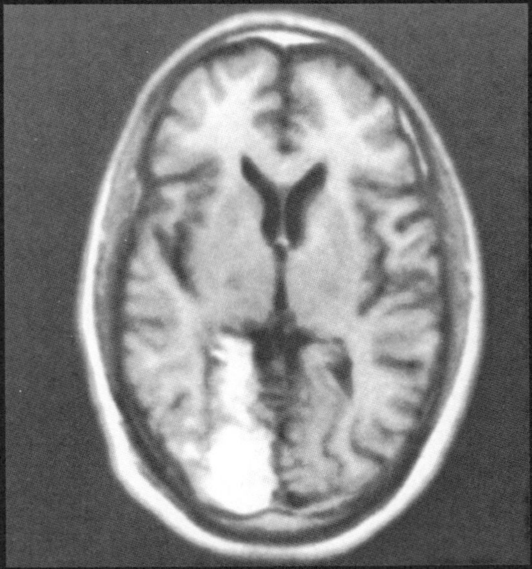

Fig. 7.69 Arteriovenous malformation; inversion recovery with gadolinium (courtesy Hammersmith Hospital)

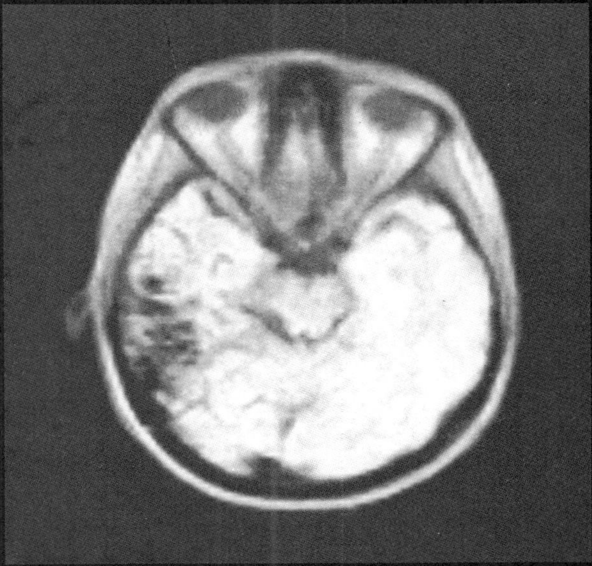

Fig. 7.70 Arteriovenous malformation; proton density; transverse

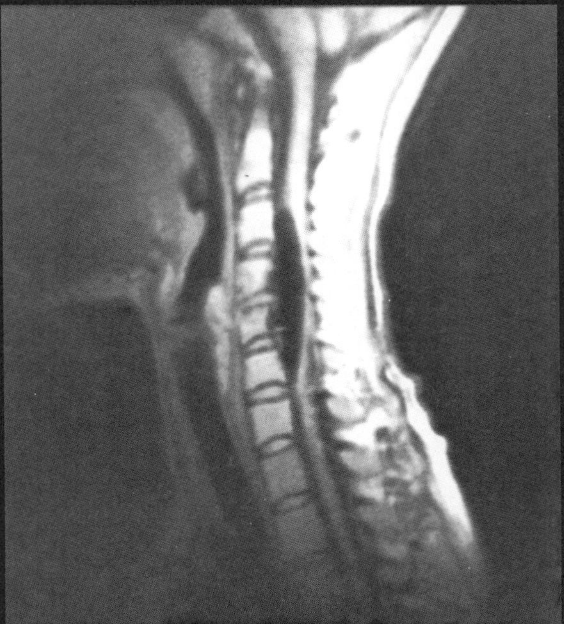

Fig. 7.71 Arteriovenous malformation in cervical spine; surface coil; sagittal (courtesy Hammersmith Hospital)

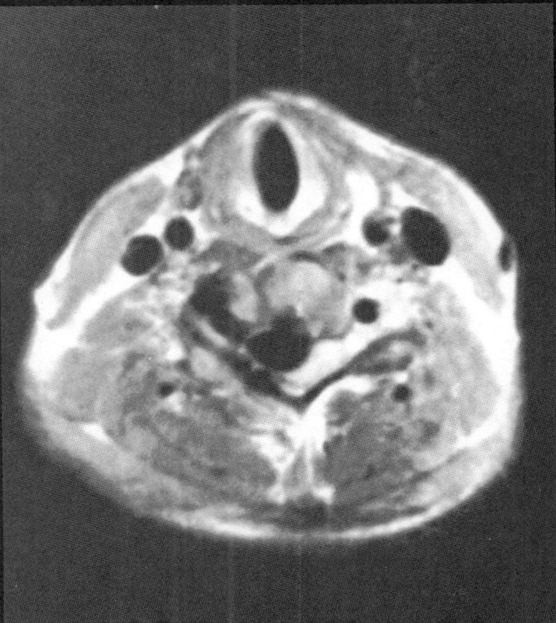

Fig. 7.72 Arteriovenous malformation in cervical spine; surface coil; transverse (courtesy Hammersmith Hospital)

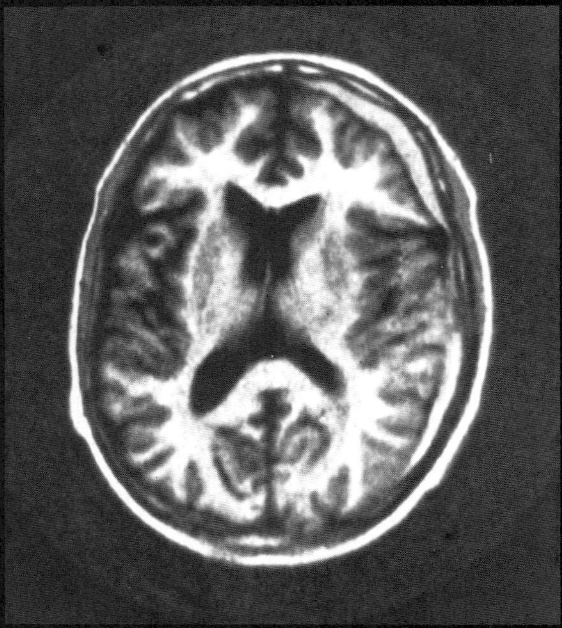

Fig. 7.73 Subdural haematoma; inversion recovery; transverse

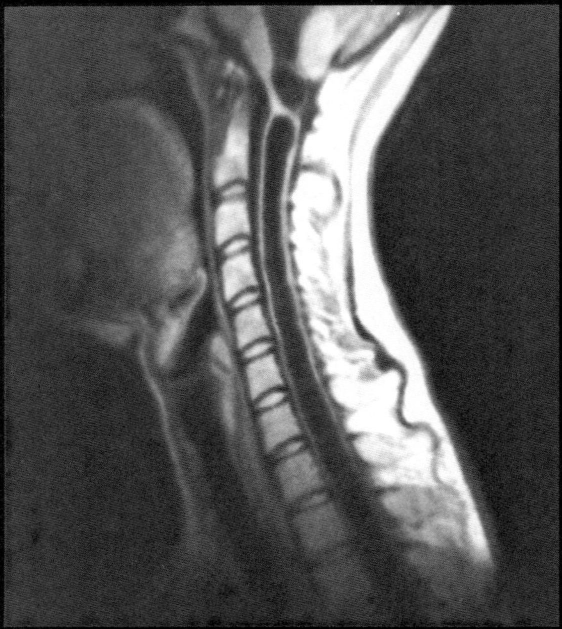

Fig. 7.74 Syringomyelia; sagittal; surface coil (courtesy Hammersmith Hospital)

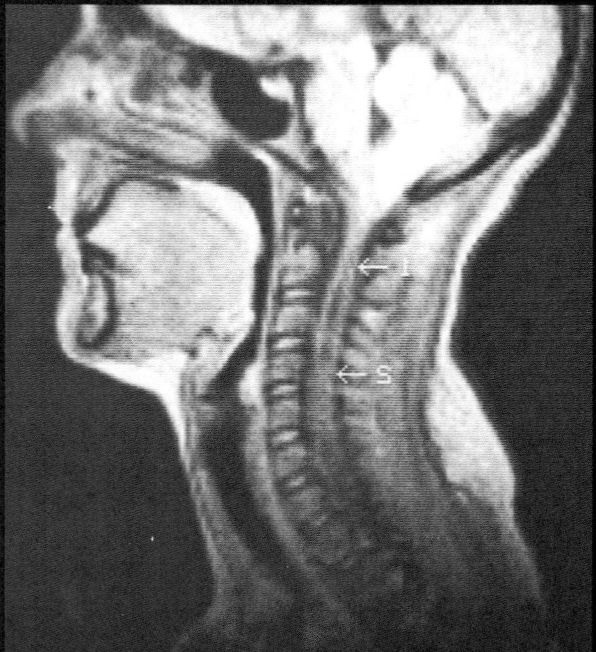

Fig. 7.75 Syrinx; proton density; sagittal

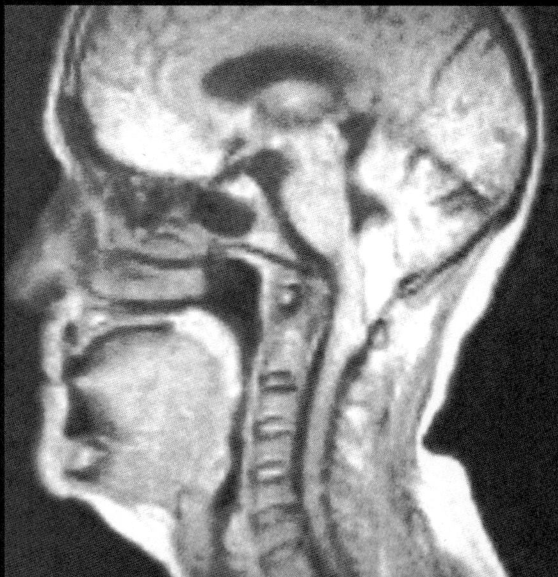

Fig. 7.76 *Arnold Chiari* malformation; proton density; sagittal

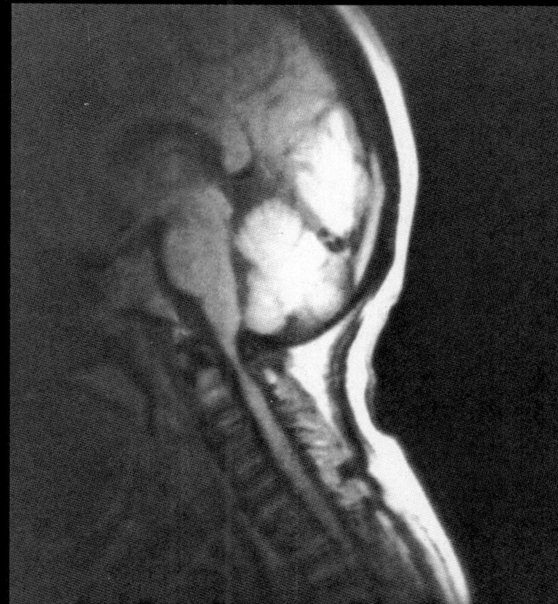

Fig. 7.77 Congenital anomaly at cranio-vertebral junction; surface coil; sagittal (courtesy Hammersmith Hospital)

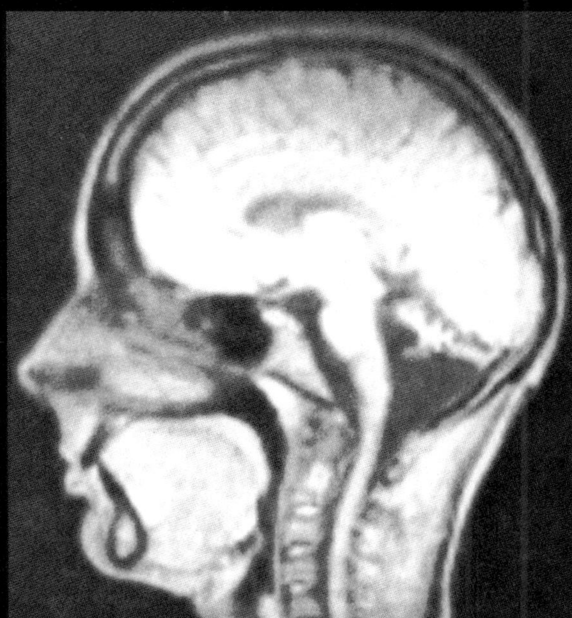

Fig. 7.78 Cerebellar hypoplasia; Proton density; Sagittal

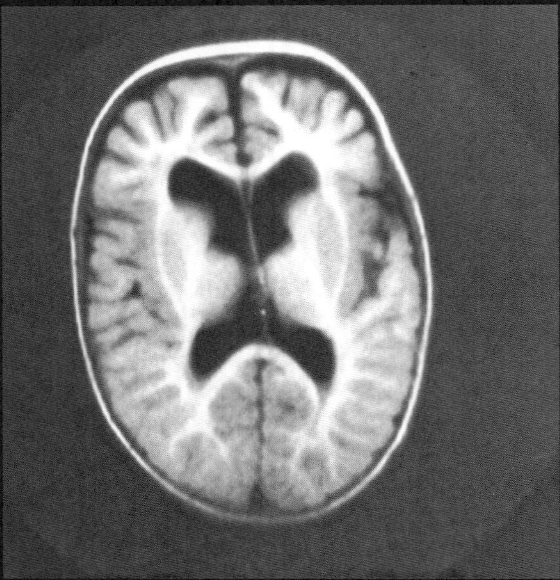

Fig. 7.79 Normal myelination; inversion recovery

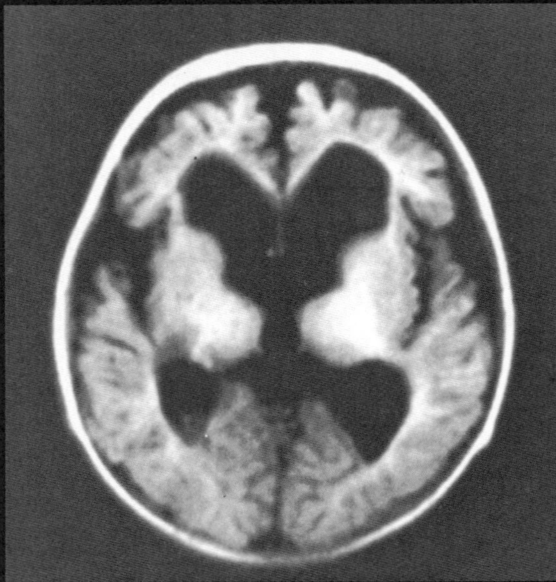

Fig. 7.80 Delayed myelination and ventricular dilatation; inversion recovery

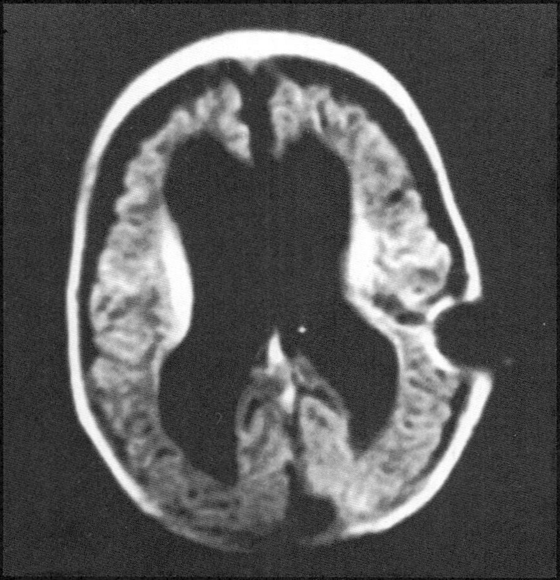

Fig. 7.81 Vetricular shunt and delayed myelination; inversion recovery

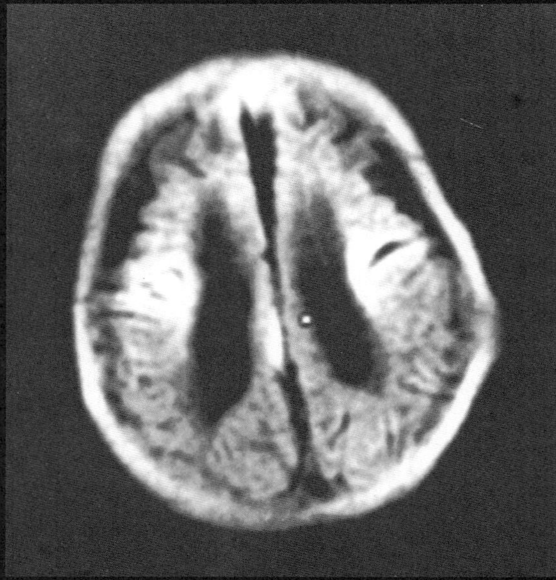

Fig. 7.82 Interhemispheric haemorrhage; inversion recovery

8

Imaging the thorax

Heart

There are some problems involved in cardiac MRI.

(1) To obtain cardiac images with the best possible resolution some method must be used to 'freeze' cardiac motion.

(2) The available contrast levels are lower in the heart than in some other parts of the body such as the brain.

(3) The examination technique is unsuited to some cardiac patients since it may involve lying flat for long periods and cardiac pacemakers are not permitted in the imaging units.

'Freezing' cardiac motion

The MR pulse sequences can be linked via an ECG to the cardiac cycle. This 'gating' allows cardiac motion to be frozen at a chosen point of the cardiac cycle at the expense of increased imaging time. If the imaging sequence is not 'gated' in this manner the resultant image is mainly of a heart in diastole since such a large percentage of the cardiac cycle is diastolic. Another solution to the problem in the future may be the echo-planar technique of Mansfield (1977). This provides 'snap-shots' of the heart since the data collection period is only about 40 ms. This effectively produces real time images of the heart but is at present limited in spatial resolution. Much work is being undertaken to improve the resolution and to increase the diameter of the patient aperture since the previous small set-up only allowed imaging of animals and babies. If implemented successfully this technique may well revolutionise cardiac MRI.

Spatial resolution of body images

There is no easy solution to the inferior spatial resolution of MR body images. In the heart it may be possible to increase the number of averages performed during data acquistion but this will increase the overall imaging time. It may also be possible to employ surface coil techniques. This will probably be limited to the investigation of the ventricles but would obviously be important if looking at myocardial ischaemia. Although several groups have demonstrated portions of the coronary arteries these have not yet been demonstrated in their full length. This type of display would be required to detect any local alterations in diameter occurring in coronary arteriosclerosis. The demonstration of even small segments of the coronary vessels may however be useful in showing patency of coronary artery graft procedures. The demonstration of the coronary vessels is further hampered by the poor spatial resolution of MR. However, it may be argued that it is not spatial resolution which is the important feature in cardiac MRI, but that the major interest should be focussed on the ability of MRI to detect alterations in tissue characteristics as may occur in myocardial ischaemia.

Contrast levels

In the brain there are several different tissue types whose relative contrasts may be altered to suit the clinical problem. This is not the case in the heart. The important structures are pericardium, myocardium and blood. The variable amount of pericardial fat normally provides good contrast if there is any pericardial pathology such as an effusion. The appearance of flowing blood depends very much on the pulse sequences employed. Rapidly flowing blood normally gives no MR signal, but flow can be highlighted in sequences such as free induction decay where flowing blood will give a high signal. Although myocardial infarction can be displayed without paramagnetic agents, recent work has demonstrated enhancement of this type of pathology after the administration of such agents and this would appear to be another area where they will be used in the future.

Examination

If a patient cannot lie supine for long then obviously he is a poor subject for what may be a long MR investigation. The examination must therefore be kept as short as possible. This can be achieved by (a) employing multiple slice techniques and perhaps bringing the patient out between different data collection sessions; (b) taking as few sections as possible by using sagittal and coronal sections to cover the area of interest instead of multiple transverse; (c) in the future by using the rapid 'echo-planar' technique. Unfortunately even doing this some patients cannot tolerate the isolated, enclosed environment of most MR systems. Pacemakers are a complete contraindication to MRI because of the magnetic fields present.

Normal cardiac anatomy

Using the common MR sequences such as inversion recovery and spin echo flowing blood within the cardiac chambers and great vessels is normally seen as zero signal contrasted against the myocardium. Without gating, the interventricular septum is routinely visualised but other structures such as the atrioventricular valves or chordae tendineae cannot be identified. Transverse sections obtained in a cephalad direction show first the ventricular cavities. Higher sections will then display the atrioventricular valves and atria followed by the origin of the great vessels and their branching. Coronal sections often show the origin of the aorta in a striking manner, and this can be followed through the chest and the point of origin of the major vessels clearly seen. Likewise, the origin of the pulmonary artery can be clearly identified and its branching in the lungs shown. The sagittal view allows the full sweep of the aorta in the thorax to be seen and also its relationship to the pulmonary artery. Since the heart lies in an oblique plane in the thorax it may be that the best way to examine the heart is to use a '3-D' or 'volume' type of acquisition and then to obtain images in any plane including the oblique.

Pathology

Even without gating it is possible to show pathological change. An assessment can be made of the size and thickness of the ventricular walls and septum and any increase in size as occurs in hypertrophic cardiomyopathy observed. These measurements compare favourably with those obtained by echocardiography and are obviously less operator-dependent. Similar changes may also be observed in the cardiomyopathies and hypertensive heart disease. Ungated images have also been used to demonstrate myocardial ischaemia and infarction in which the abnormal areas are characterised by elevation of the relaxation times and a little increase in the proton density relative to normal myocardium in the acute stage. Such changes may not be seen in very early infarcts which are less than 3 hours old and much work has been performed to improve the detection of infarction using paramagnetic agents (early workers used manganese but more recent research has employed gadolinium) and their use, coupled with gating, has greatly improved the delineation of infarcts. Both inversion recovery and spin echo sequences, i.e. T_1 and T_2 weighted images have been used to successfully demonstrate infarction. As well as the demonstration of recent infarction it is also possible to show the late effects and complications of infarction, for example localised areas of ventricular wall thinning, thrombus formation, ventricular aneurysms, etc.

(Figs 8.1 to 8.5).

By comparing gated images of the left ventricle obtained at end systole and end diastole it is possible to estimate the approximate ejection fraction. Pericardial effusions are easily demonstrated by MRI and may be seen in some cases where there is no other evidence (such as echocardiography) of their existence. Cardiac MRI has been used to demonstrate the anatomical abnormalities present in congenital heart disease but its precise role in this field requires much more work.

Mediastinum

The mediastinum is arguably the region of the thorax where MRI will find its greatest clinical application. There are several reasons for this.

(1) On most MR sequences flowing blood gives zero signal and this provides great contrast between the vascular hilar structures and their surrounding anatomy of fat, lymph nodes and lung; the air-filled bronchi are normally seen as zero signal branching structures but if there is any doubt then the pulse sequences can be altered to increase the signal from blood which will then be contrasted against the bronchi whose signal will remain zero.

(2) The pulse sequences can be altered to highlight pathological change.

(3) Coronal and sagittal sections allow very accurate anatomical localisation of pathology to be made and these sections, particularly the coronal, are very useful in defining the relationships of hilar and mediastinal masses to their neighbouring vessels.

Normal mediastinal anatomy

The anatomy displayed on transverse sections closely parallels that visible on contrast enhanced CT with the vascular structures (usually zero signal) contrasted against the intermediate signal of nodes and high signal fat. The ultimate resolution obtainable depends on whether gating is employed. Respiratory and cardiac can be used. Respiratory gating is advisable if looking at the lung fields, and cardiac gating is useful when looking at the mediastinum. The best spatial resolution is achieved when both forms of gating are employed, but as each increases the imaging time then using both may make the investigation too long, bearing in mind that some of the patients may suffer from dyspnoea and be unsuitable for a protracted MR examination. The ultimate resolution of the transverse MR image is inferior to good quality CT and particular care must be taken if looking for small lesions in the lung fields. Coronal sections are, in combination with transverse sections, useful in the clarification of anatomical relations in the lung apices, diaphragmatic regions and the hila.

Pathology

Again most forms of pathology demonstrate elevated relaxation times. It is impossible to accurately predict the tissue type by the relaxation times, but it has been observed that lymphomatous tissue has a relaxation time which although elevated is not as high as bronchogenic or metastatic neoplasm. It has also been observed that there is an overlap between neoplasia and infection and it is therefore impossible to predict for example if an abnormal node is abnormal due to neoplasia or secondary infection. The behaviour of the signal from fat with alteration of the pulse parameters is very important. Fat has a short T_1 but a long T_2. Most pathology displays increase in both these relaxation times. Sequences with a short *TR*—that is, T_1-dependent—will display most contrast between pathology (long T_1) and fat (short T_1). These sequences will, however, give a poorer overall signal to noise than sequences with longer *TR*. If possible the examination should be carried out using two different pulse parameters, the first to optimise the pathological contrast and the second to obtain an image with better signal to noise and therefore better resolution. In summary, the short *TR* sequences emphasise T_1 differences and so give more pathological input and the T_2 images (long *TR* spin echo) give the better anatomical detail. It has been shown that cardiac gating is useful in assessing masses in the anterior mediastinum and hilum, but is not a significant improvement in masses in the relatively fixed superior mediastinum.

Lung

The diagnosis of pulmonary parenchymal abnormalities has received little attention in MR research. There are a few reasons for this.

(1) As previously stated the ultimate spatial resolution of body MR is inferior to that obtainable in the head.

(2) Calcification cannot be visualised and therefore it may be impossible to distinguish benign from malignant lesions using this important sign.

(3) Respiratory and perhaps cardiac gating would be required to increase the image quality to enable small lesions to be identified and this would increase the imaging time to perhaps unacceptable levels.

At the present time therefore there is no definite area in the lung fields where MR is superior to CT—in fact it is probably the converse at present. However, in the future we may see improvements with altered pulse sequences to allow total lung imaging in a shorter time and the use of gaseous paramagnetic agents may allow more accurate tissue characterisation. In general, most pulmonary pathology displays elevated relaxation times with the unfortunate overlap of neoplasia and infection. It is possible to differentiate post-radiation fibrosis from tumour recurrence since fibrosis, although displaying an elevated T_2 the rise is less than that observed in tumour. The lung following pulmonary embolism has a shorter T_1 than normal. This fact, coupled with paramagnetic gases, will perhaps allow for magnetic ventilation perfusion scans in the future. Pleural thickening is characterised by displaying a relatively short T_1. Pleural fluid has a low proton density and a long T_1. T_1 measurement may allow for characterisation of effusions since T_1 falls as the proton concentration of an effusion rises. After the rapid infusion of large quantities of fluid (about 2 litres) both the T_1 and proton density of the lung rise indicating an increase in extravascular lung water, and this fact may be useful in making non-invasive assessments of lung water. The MR signal from the lungs is mainly derived from the lung parenchyma and not the vasculature as is the case in CT. This signal is also gravity-dependent with more signal being observed from the dependent lung. (Figs 8.6, 8.7 and 8.8).

Breast

Advantages of MRI in imaging the breast

(1) If MRI can be shown to be a useful and sensitive technique in the investigation of the breast, it would be a very attractive imaging modality due to its lack of non ionising radiation.

(2) Another advantage is the potential of more accurate tissue characterisation.

Disadvantages of MRI in imaging the breast

(1) The fact that MRI cannot detect calcification, particularly the microcalcification which is an important indicator of breast disease, is a significant handicap.

(2) The ranges of tissue contrast present in the breast may make the detection of pathology difficult.

(3) The long time required for an MR breast examination makes it unlikely the MRI could be used as a screening procedure.

(4) A breast coil is required to obtain the highest quality images. This normally provides an image of one breast at a time thus further increasing the examination time if one wants to image both breasts for comparative purposes.

(5) The research performed to date still appears to display an unfortunate overlap in MR parameters and different types of pathology.

Normal

The normal breast is composed of variable amounts of fatty tissue, connective stroma and glandular elements. The short T_1 fat gives a high signal on inversion recovery images and provides contrast with the stromal elements and glandular tissue which has a higher T_1 than the fatty components. The optimum method for the examination of the breast is with a purpose designed breast coil into which the breast is positioned. One important point which must be remembered when using these coils is that they provide only a localised view and do not therefore image important areas such as the axilla or the region of the internal mammary drainage where metastases may be found.

Pathology

Most researchers working in the field of breast MRI have used short *TR*, *TE* sequences as an intitial 'scout' sequence. Any abnormality seen can then be re-examined using longer *TR*, *TE* sequences. Inversion recovery sequences may also be used. The problems in the choice of sequence arise from the difficulty in differentiating long T_1 pathology in the region of breast tissue which also has a moderately long T_1 and in separating long T_2 lesions from long T_2 fat. As in other regions of the body it may be wise to examine the breast using two different pulse sequences to avoid missing a lesion due to these difficulties. Malignant disease displays elevation in relaxation times but there may be some overlap in these times, and in those seen in normal breast tissue especially close to the nipple and some benign conditions such as fibroadenomata. In general however, benign conditions have shorter relaxation times than malignant ones. Breast cysts have very long relaxation times and are usually easily recognised. Even large areas of calcification will not be seen by MRI.

Due to the many difficulties described in MRI of the breast it may be that MRI will not be used as an initial screening examination but its ultimate role may be as an adjunct to other investigations such as mammography where it may provide more information as to the nature of a suspicious area in the breast. Another area where MRI may be particularly useful is in screening for metastatic disease in the axilla and the internal mammary drainage area both being areas which are not well visualised by other techniques.

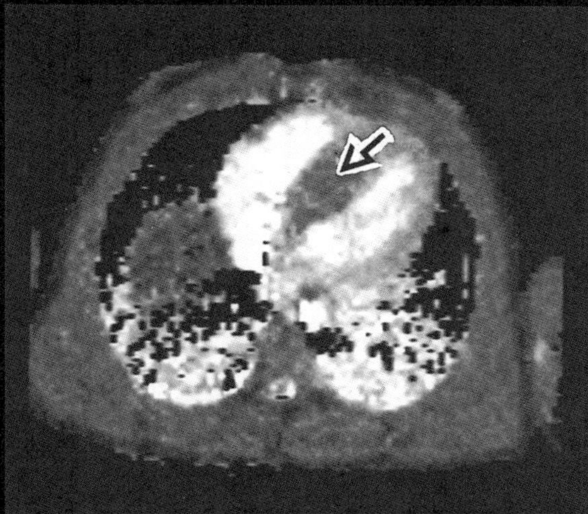

Fig. 8.1 Hypertrophic cardiomyopathy illustrating septum.

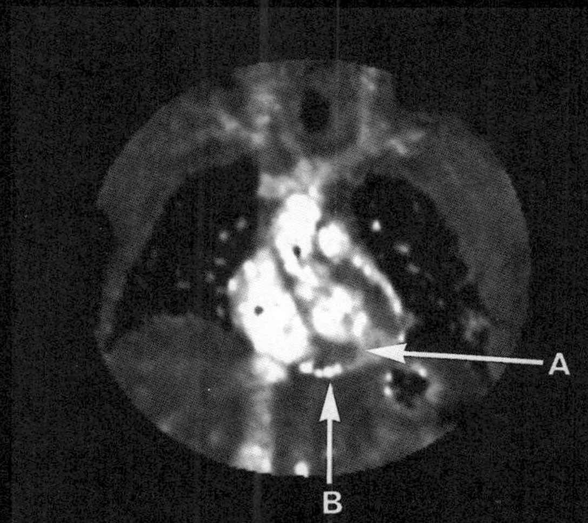

Fig. 8.2 Calculated T_1 image, obtained with cardiac gating, shows high signal from a recent infarct in the left ventricle (A). A small pericardial effusion (B) is also seen

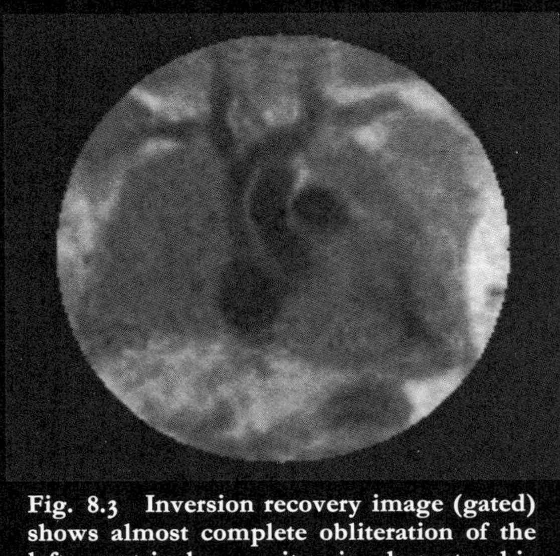

Fig. 8.3 Inversion recovery image (gated) shows almost complete obliteration of the left ventricular cavity in hypertrophic cardiomyopathy

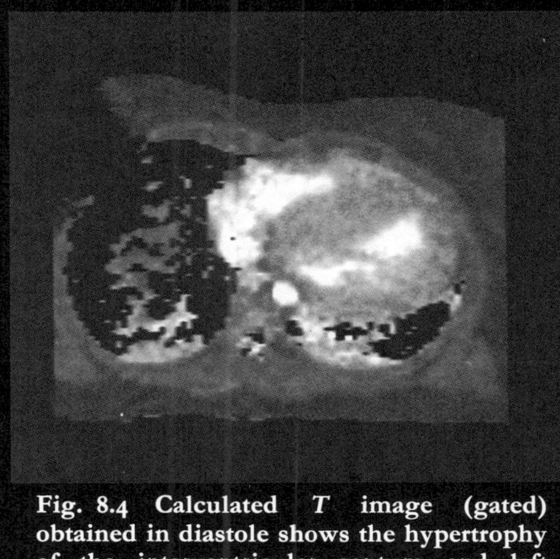

Fig. 8.4 Calculated T image (gated) obtained in diastole shows the hypertrophy of the interventricular septum and left ventricle in hypertrophic cardiomyopathy

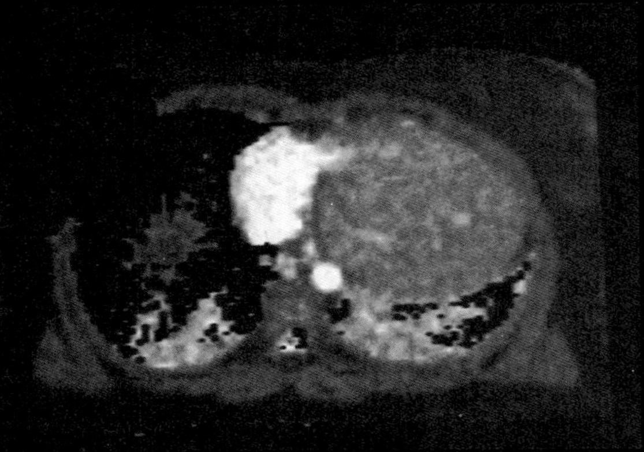

Fig. 8.5 Calculated T_1 image (gated) is of the same subject shown in Fig. 8.4 but obtained in systole. This demonstrates the virtual obliteration of the left ventricular cavity which may occur in this condition

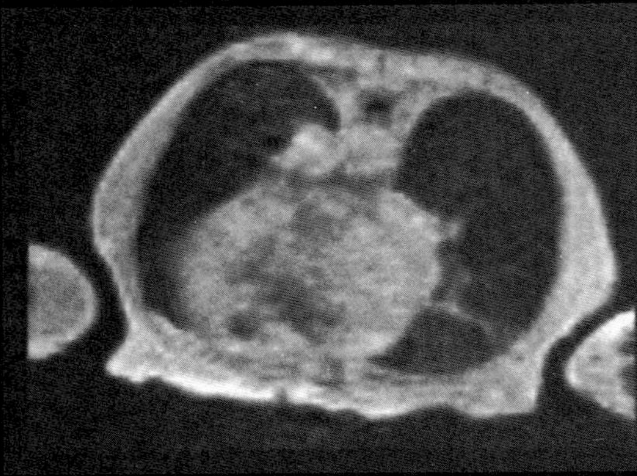

Fig. 8.6 Pericardial cyst; proton density

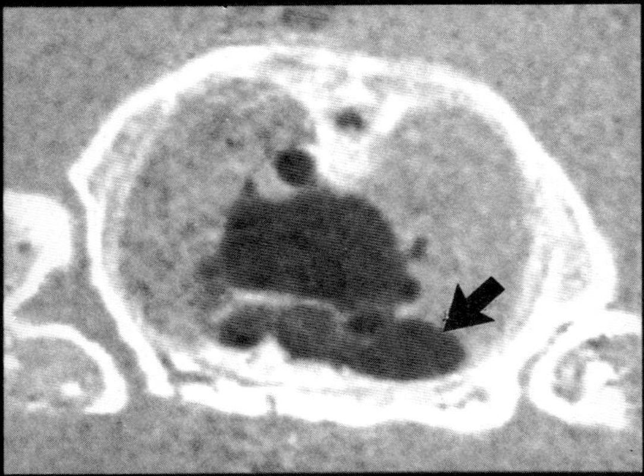

Fig. 8.7 Pericardial cyst; inversion recovery illustrating the position of the cyst

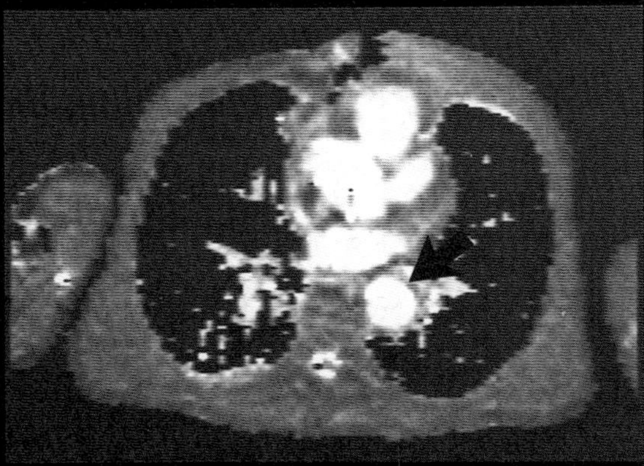

Fig. 8.8 Thoracic aortic dissection; calculated T_1. Arrow points to flap in the dissected descending aorta

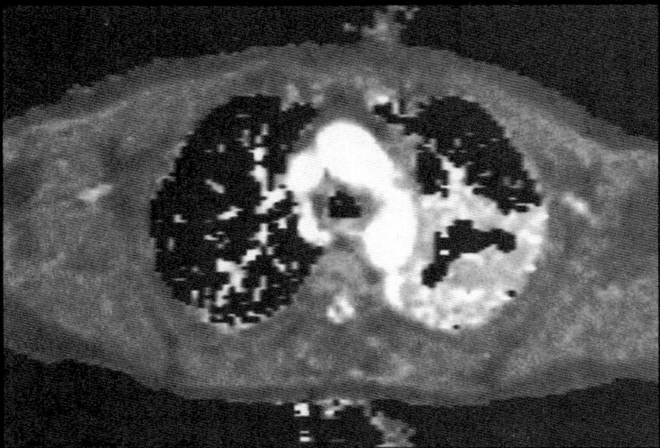

Fig. 8.9 Cavitating bronchogenic carcinoma; calculated T_1

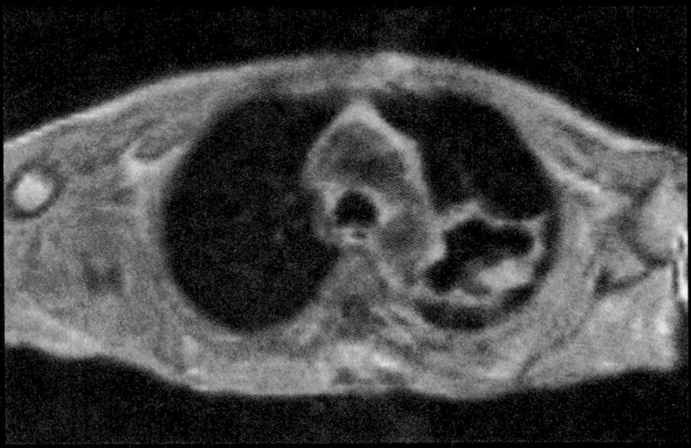

Fig. 8.10 Cavitating bronchogenic carcinoma; proton density

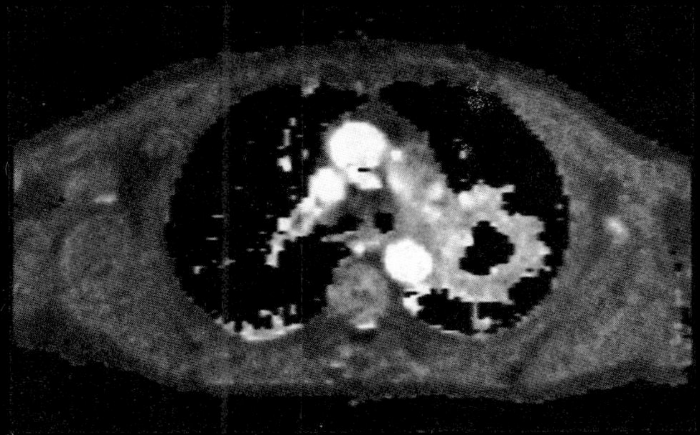

Fig. 8.11 Mediastinal involvement by bronchogenic carcinoma

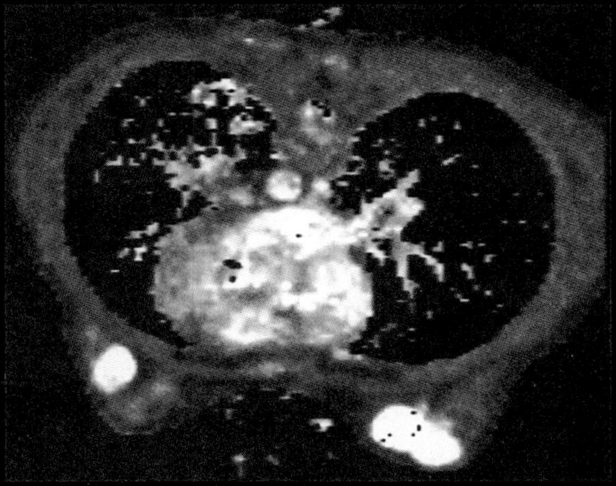

Fig. 8.12 Breast cysts; calculated T_1

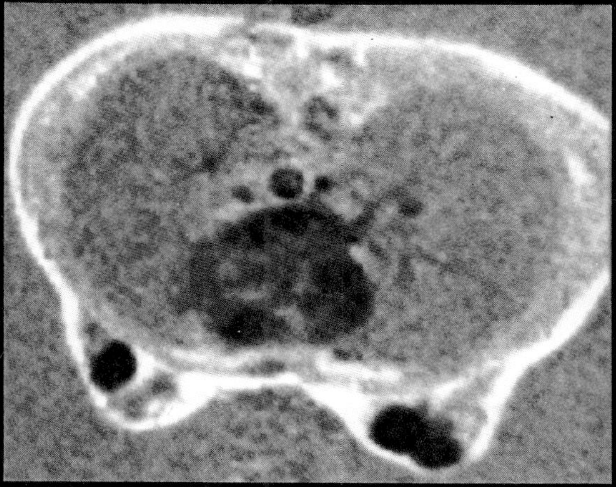

Fig. 8.13 Breast cysts; inversion recovery

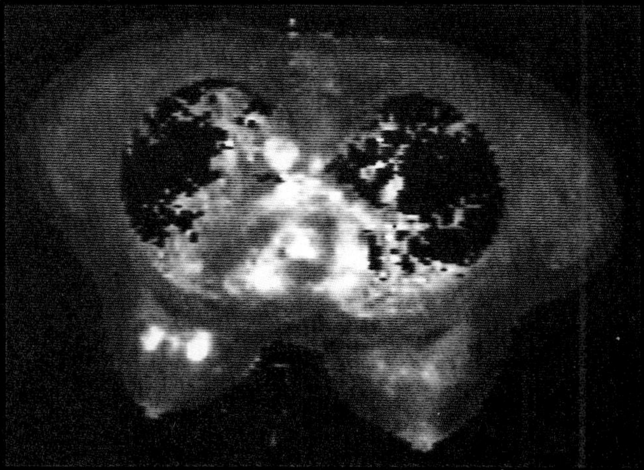

Fig. 8.14 Breast cysts; calculated T_1

9

Imaging the abdomen and pelvis

General

Inversion recovery images are useful in defining normal anatomy and are particularly useful in highlighting the T_1 differences between the short T_1 of fat and an immediately adjacent organ with a higher T_1 such as the kidney. As with CT fat provides excellent contrast in abdominal MRI and this can be highlighted by alteration of the pulse sequence variables. Short *TR* inversion recovery sequences will highlight T_1 differences and this can be useful in defining the anatomy around organs surrounded by fat such as the kidney. Short *TR*, *TE* spin echo sequences will give a higher signal to noise ratio and spatial resolution and may be useful when trying to identify small lesions. One must be careful when using longer *TR*, *TE* spin echo sequences in the abdomen, since intra-abdominal fat has a long T_2 and will therefore give a high signal leading to problems of contrast.

Advantages of MRI in imaging the abdomen

(1) The pulse sequence variables can be optimised to suit the clinical problem.

(2) There are no artefacts from some substances which pose problems in CT such as dense barium, the air-fluid interface in the stomach and metallic prostheses which cause streak artefacts in the pelvis.

(3) There is 'natural' MR contrast between blood vessels and adjacent anatomy such as lymph nodes.

(4) The multiplanar facility provides accurate localisation of intra-abdominal pathology.

(5) Abdominal MRI is not as dependent on the skill of the operator as is the case with ultrasound and, unlike ultrasound, excess bowel gas does not degrade the quality of the examination; in some cases it may actually improve it by increasing the contrast between gas-filled bowel loops and adjacent anatomy such as pancreas and lymph nodes.

Disadvantages of MRI in imaging the abdomen

(1) There is some degradation of the abdominal MR image due to respiratory and transmitted cardiac motion particularly in the upper abdomen, and therefore gating is required to provide the best quality images.

(2) As yet there is no readily available bowel-opacifying agent; loops of small bowel containing fluid with long relaxation times may cause problems when adjacent to lymph nodes, pancreas and in the pelvis. Ferric chloride has been used to 'opacify' the stomach and upper small bowel but cannot be used routinely. Fatty compounds such as milk and ice cream have also been tried with limited success. A very useful ploy when concerned with the upper abdomen is to paralyse the bowel with an intravenous injection of a relaxant such as glucagon and also to distend the bowel by giving the patient effervescent gas tablets. This outlines the bowel, particularly the duodenum, very well and may eliminate the problem of differentiating upper small bowel from pancreas.

(3) The limited spatial resolution compared to CT is a handicap when trying to assess minor degrees of lymphadenopathy.

Liver

Normal anatomy

The anatomical features displayed on transverse MR sections are very similar to those seen on CT. There is no streaking from the air-fluid interface in the stomach. There is a little loss of resolution if the acquisition is ungated and this should be employed when looking for small lesions. Coronal sections show the vascular anatomy adjacent to the liver very well, and in particular the hepatic veins can often be seen draining into the inferior vena cava on coronal MR examinations of the upper abdomen. The coronal and sagittal planes identify the liver in relation to the diaphragm and are useful in assessing the extent of subphrenic and subhepatic pathology. The portal venous system can be differentiated from intrahepatic biliary radicles in two ways: either by looking at a 'routine' saturation recovery image with a sufficiently long *TR* so that hepatic blood vessels are not seen, but bile ducts are seen as regions of zero signal, particularly when they start to dilate. Alternatively, if the *TR* is reduced then the portal venous system will be seen to give a higher signal due to the increase in signal from flowing blood observed with these sequences.

Pathology

The choice of pulse sequence is critical. Unlike other organs such as the brain where there is a wide range of tissue contrast available, in the liver this range is much more restricted, and therefore lesions may easily be missed if an inappropriate pulse sequence is chosen (see Fig. 3.13, p. 34). It would therefore appear sensible to examine the liver using at least two different pulse sequence parameters. Standard saturation recovery sequences are an insensitive method in examining the liver since hepatic pathology shows little difference in proton density and may be invisible on this type of image. More T_1 weighted images such as saturation recovery sequences with a short *TR* are sensitive to a wide range of disease. Hepatic tissue has a characteristic T_1 value and measurements of this may be useful in trying to assess hepatic pathology. Prolonged relaxation times occur in hepatitis, cirrhosis, neoplasms, atrophy, infarction, obstruction and infection. In cholecystitis the T_1 of liver and bile increases. Only a small elevation in the relaxation times is observed in hepatitis and cirrhosis while neoplastic conditions are associated with much more pronounced elevations of these times. In cirrhosis the degree of elevation of T_1 may be a sensitive indicator of the severity of disease. The elevation of T_1 is slightly less in hepatomas than in other types of malignancy, but it is not possible to predict the type of malignancy from a measured relaxation time. The fluid in most hepatic cysts has a very long T_1; this will fall due to the short T_1 of blood if there has been recent haemorrhage. Shortening of the relaxation times occur in haemochromatosis and haemosiderosis but despite the short T_1 of fat, the T_1 of liver in fatty infiltration has often been observed to be still within the normal range although at the lower end. T_2 may prove to be a more sensitive parameter for assessing fatty infiltration. The recently developed technique of simple proton spectroscopic imaging appears to be more able to detect fatty infiltration in the liver. The deposition of paramagnetic substances such as iron and copper in the liver cause an overall decrease in hepatic relaxation times. This effect is seen in Wilson's disease (copper), haemochromatosis and haemosiderosis (iron). There may be some clues to different types of pathology, such as a necrotic centre in some tumours or a draining vein in a haemangioma. The exceptionally long T_1 of a simple cyst should make this diagnosis simple. Biliary calculi are not seen unless they are very large.

Dilute bile has relatively long T_1 and T_2 values which are seen to decrease as bile is concentrated in the gall bladder. Thus, it would appear that MRI could be used to assess gall bladder function either by making T_1 or T_2 measurements, or by comparing signal intensities of bile in fasting and non fasting states, since for example, shortening of T_1 would lead to an increase in signal intensity on the same MR pulse sequence.

Spleen

The relaxation times of normal splenic tissue are higher than those of normal liver. There has been little work to date regarding MRI of the spleen. Various tumours such as lymphoma and metastases have been demonstrated in the spleen. The future of MRI in the investigation of the spleen may lie in its potential to assess splenic involvement by lymphoma. MRI has not yet been demonstrated to be particularly useful in the investigation of the lymphomas. There appears to be little difference in the MR characteristics of lymphomatous nodes and nodes containing metastatic tumour. Lymph nodes have a longer T_1 than fat and are shown well by short *TR* sequences. It is also possible to assess the age of a splenic thrombus by MRI since a more recent blood collection will have a shorter T_1 (Figs. 9.1 to 9.13). The relaxation times of the spleen often rise in portal hypertension perhaps suggesting splenic oedema and venous congestion.

Pancreas

It may be difficult to identify the normal pancreas particularly if there is little intra-abdominal fat since it may appear very similar to adjacent bowel loops and lymph nodes. However when it is involved by infection or neoplasm its relaxation times prolong and this usually provides contrast between it and surrounding anatomy. However the prolongation of relaxation times may be only slight and often one has to rely, as in CT, on morphological criteria for the identification of pancreatic neoplasia. One tumour which consistently appears to give significantly higher signal than normal pancreas is the islet cell type. In infective processes the pancreas may appear to be surrounded by a collection of very long relaxation time fluid. Neoplasms elevate pancreatic relaxation times more than infection. Enlarged nodes, particularly in the coeliac region, may appear to merge with the abnormal pancreas due to their proximity and to their similar MR appearance when abnormal. Pancreatic MRI should improve with the use of MR bowel labelling, respiratory gating and perhaps by the more routine use of paramagnetic agents. At present, if in doubt, it may be useful to give the subject some gas and glucagon as described under 'disadvantages'. This will establish the position of the pancreas in almost every instance and eliminates the contrast problem of bowel fluid with long relaxation times. A final disadvantage of MRI in pancreatic imaging that must be mentioned is the inability to detect small areas of calcification.

Adrenals

The adrenals are visualised in a similar fashion to CT but MRI may prove to have at least two advantages over CT.

(1) Even a small amount of fat adjacent to the adrenals can provide great contrast between this fat and the adrenal; this contrast can be emphasised by using T_1-weighted sequences such as those with a short *TR* repetition rate.

(2) The zero MR signal from flowing blood will permit distinction between adjacent vascular structures and the adrenal which may cause confusion, particularly on the right.

Even though the spatial resolution of MR is at present inferior to CT this may be improved in small anatomical regions such as the adrenals by using surface coils and by increasing the number of averages performed during data acquisition. This is particularly relevant to adrenal MRI since the adrenals occupy a small anatomical area, and therefore more time can profitably be spent improving resolution by signal averaging. Respiratory gating may also improve the image quality.

Pathology

Adrenal pathology is relatively easily assessed but as yet the changes shown have been non-specific. In hyperplasia, although MR like CT can show enlargement at a relatively late stage, it is hoped that in the future earlier stages of hyperplasia will be detected by analysing the adrenal relaxation times. Neoplasms and infections are characterised by elevated relaxation times. Adrenal haemorrhage is characterised by areas of shortened relaxation times (Fig. 9.19).

Kidneys

In the kidneys the presence of fat in the perirenal tissues and renal hilum provides contrast between these structures and renal tissue. Due to the short T_1 of fat this differentiation is accentuated by using short *TR* pulse sequences. The normal renal cortex has a shorter T_1 than the medulla and therefore appears of higher signal intensity on inversion recovery sequences. This corticomedullary differentiation is accentuated by decreasing *TR* and is also dependent on the degree of hydration. In a state of diuresis it is accentuated. Other anatomical features which can be distinguised easily are urine in the collecting systems and renal pelvis, which is characterised by its long T_1 and T_2 values. These long relaxation times allow a dilated renal pelvis and ureter to be differentiated from adjacent structures such as nodes and blood vessels. If a multiple echo spin echo sequence is employed the signal intensity of urine on successive echoes will increase relative to the surrounding anatomy due to the long T_2 of urine. The renal vasculature will be displayed as zero signal on most MR sequences due to the flow phenomenon and therefore the vessels are easily traced to the inferior vena cava and aorta. This appearance of the vessels can be used to assess spread of renal neoplasms, whose presence within the renal vein can be quickly and confidently shown without venography or arteriography.

Pathology

MR features of renal pathology are:

(1) Loss of the corticomedullary differentiation.
(2) Focal or diffuse alterations in relaxation times.
(3) Alterations in contour.
(4) Evidence of renal obstruction and hydronephrosis.

Relaxation times rise in most forms of renal pathology with the exception of haemorrhage where the abnormal area is characterised by having a shorter T_1 than surrounding renal tissue. Of particular interest is the fact that MR may be able to differentiate tubular necrosis from rejection. This would obviously be of particular relevance in the case of renal transplantation. In necrosis the kidneys are swollen, there is some loss of corticomedullary differentiation and the relaxation times are moderately elevated. In rejection similar features are observed but the changes are more severe. The kidneys are seen to be more swollen, there is complete loss of corticomedullary differentiation and the relaxation times are elevated to levels up to three times those observed in necrosis. In early obstruction dilation of the renal collecting system can be seen, and the T_1 of renal cortex is seen to rise with continuing obstruction until it approaches that of the medulla. The T_1 of renal medulla does not appear to rise in obstruction and the corticomedullary distinction is eventually lost. This assessment of renal T_1 may therefore be useful in determining the 'age' of an obstructed kidney. In renal infection not only are the relaxation times elevated in a diffuse manner throughout the kidney but there is also loss of the corticomedullary differentiation. These T_1 and T_2 elevations which occur in renal infection are sensitive but not specific as are the changes which occur in renal neoplasms.

The changes in neoplasm allow for identification of the presence of a focal lesion, but as in other areas of the body it it impossible to predict the histological variety on the basis of relaxation time data. It must be remembered that not all renal carcinomas have prolonged relaxation times. This should not detract from the use of MR in the staging of renal malignancy due to the following:

(1) The ability to assess the extent of the tumour particularly when sagittal and coronal sections are obtained in addition to transverse.

(2) The ease and reliability of demonstrating renal vein involvement.

(3) The potential to demonstrate spread to adjacent lymph nodes. Short *TR* sequences will accentuate differences between cortex and medulla and between lymph nodes and fat.

The inability to demonstrate calcification is a major shortcoming of renal MRI. A consequence of this is the inability of MR to demonstrate small renal calculi. Renal cysts are readily shown by MR both by alteration of contour and also by the cyst fluid which has very high T_1 and T_2 values. It is also possible to demonstrate haemorrhage within cysts since this will shorten the relaxation times of the cyst fluid. MR can be used to differentiate between a cyst and fat in the region of the renal sinus. This is an area which can pose problems for both ultrasound and CT but these two entities can be differentiated easily by using MR due to the very short T_1 of fat and the very long T_1 of cyst fluid (Figs. 9.20 to 9.24).

Pelvis

Male

The bladder is an easily identifiable landmark in the pelvis and pelvic MRI is preferably performed with a comfortably full bladder. Urine in the bladder is easily identified by its long T_1 and T_2 values. The multiplanar facility of MRI is particularly useful in the pelvis and can provide a rapid and accurate delineation of the bladder base, prostate and seminal vesicles. These are all areas which are often not well demonstrated by CT. Blood vessels are easily distinguished from adjacent anatomy by the MR flow phenomenon. Pelvic lymph nodes are characterised by possessing rather longer relaxation times than adjacent pelvic viscera and musculature. Pelvic fat provides contrast and this can be accentuated by using short *TR* sequences.

MRI of the prostate is relatively simple. The sagittal and coronal planes are to be preferred since they provide a precise delineation of the gland. The sagittal plane shows the relation of the gland to the bladder base very clearly. The coronal plane demonstrates the lateral margins of the gland. Most prostatic pathology is characterised by elevation of the relaxation times. It was initially thought that measurement of MR parameters, in particular T_1 would provide confident differentiation between prostatitis and prostatic neoplasm, but further work has shown some overlap in the relaxation times of these two conditions, perhaps due to the coexistence of infection and neoplasm. The main application of MR in the prostate would appear to be in the staging of prostatic neoplasm. This can be demonstrated even when it is still limited within the prostate. The extension of disease outside the gland is accurately visualised by using the sagittal and coronal planes. Extension into the seminal vesicles can be seen and the sagittal plane shows involvement of the bladder base particularly well. Involvement of the seminal vesicles is demonstrated by referring to the normal MR appearance of these structures where their wall can be differentiated from fluid within them by highlighting the signal from the long T_2 fluid by using a long *TE* spin echo sequence. Pathological involvement is shown by noting a difference in the signal intensity when compared with its neighbour and also by noting any asymmetry. This comparison is again facilitated by the multiplanar capability of MR. In the bladder the main application appears to be in the multiplanar imaging of neoplasms as well as the superior demonstration of lesions close to the base of the bladder. Again this is an area where CT may run into problems but where sagittal and coronal MR images clearly delineate the extent of disease. Bladder tumours cause a focal increase in relaxation times whereas benign bladder wall hypertrophy secondary to low-grade outlet obstruction produces an increase in relaxation and signal intensity, on spin echo sequences, throughout the entire bladder wall (Figs. 9.25 to 9.27).

Female

The striated muscle of the pelvic musculature has a slightly longer T_1 than the smooth muscle of the uterus. This permits differentiation between these two tissues and this can be accentuated by altering *TR*. Another important feature is the difference in T_2 which exists between myometrium and endometrium. There is virtually no difference in the T_1 of these two tissues, and therefore short *TR* sequences will not demonstrate any difference. However, by employing long *TR*, long *TE* sequences the separation of the two tissue types becomes more obvious. The optimum MR sequences in the female pelvis would therefore be those with long *TR* and long *TE* since these will not only provide the greatest contrast between uterine and pelvic muscles, but also between endometrium and myometrium. These sequences are also the most useful when imaging the cervix and vagina. The vagina is clearly seen extending upwards and backwards between bladder and rectum.

The sagittal plane is the optimum plane for the demonstration of the vagina and adjacent anatomy. Long *TR* sequences demonstrate a difference in signal between the uterus and vagina, due to the longer T_1 of the vagina, which therefore appears of lower intensity than uterus on long *TR* sequences. Visualisation of pathology in the female genitourinary system is facilitated by using the multiplanar facility and most forms of pathology are characterised by an elevation of relaxation times. One exception to this is endometriosis where the implants are often observed to be of shorter T_1 than other pelvic mass lesions. This can be explained by the fact that they may contain blood with a short T_1. MRI would therefore appear to be very useful not only in identifying these deposits, but may also be used to assess their response to therapy. Ovarian cysts are usually of high signal intensity due to the presence of long T_1, T_2 fluid but this may not be the case if haemorrhage has occurred into them. A major problem exists in the assessment of the post-operative female pelvis where it may be very difficult to differentiate between fibrosis, either from radiotherapy or surgery, recurrent tumour and bowel loops which may be adherent and bound to pelvic organs. This is an area where reliable bowel labelling is urgently required; so also is considerably more clinical experience, since this is also an area where CT faces problems, and where MR may eventually prove of value.

There has to date been only limited experience with MRI in pregnancy; however, it is clear that it may have a role in the future. It can be used as a method, employing non-ionising radiation, of obtaining accurate pelvimetric measurements. The sagittal plane allows a measurement to be obtained of the anteroposterior pelvic diameter and transverse dimensions are obtained from transverse sections. If a multiple slice technique is employed then these dimensions can be obtained at varying levels in the pelvis. Other potential applications include the investigation of the 'fetus at risk' where there may be MR features in the placenta which will allow identification of a maternal or fetal cause. Fetuses with growth retardation show a diminution in body fat which is easily shown by MR; fetal abnormalities such as hydrocephalus can also be demonstrated *in utero*.

MR techniques may be particularly useful in cases where an ultrasound examination has been less than satisfactory for example in cases of oligohydramnios or obesity. The sagittal plane also allows for a very rapid and accurate assessment of the cervix and could be used to investigate such things as failure of ripening, dystocia, slow cervimetric progress and incompetence.

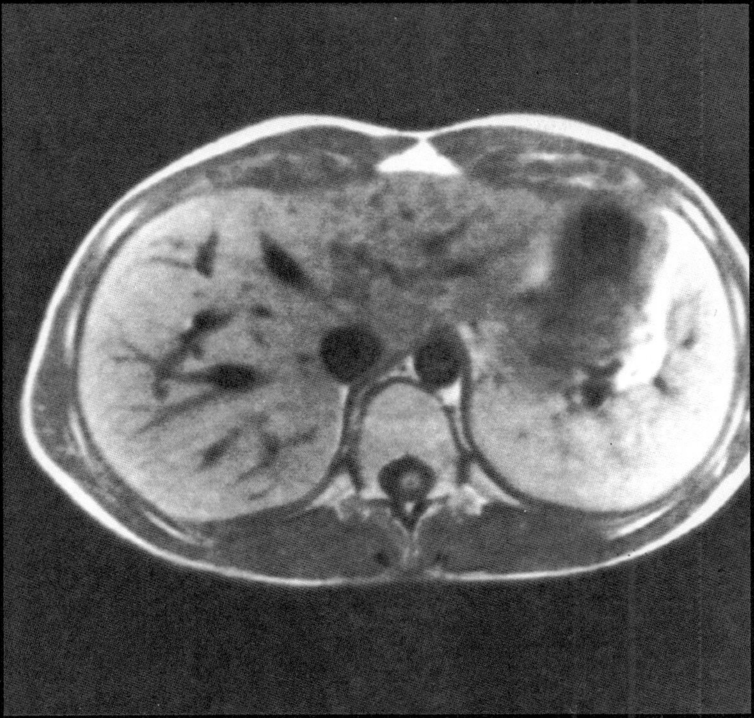

Fig. 9.1 Normal liver (courtesy Hammersmith Hospital)

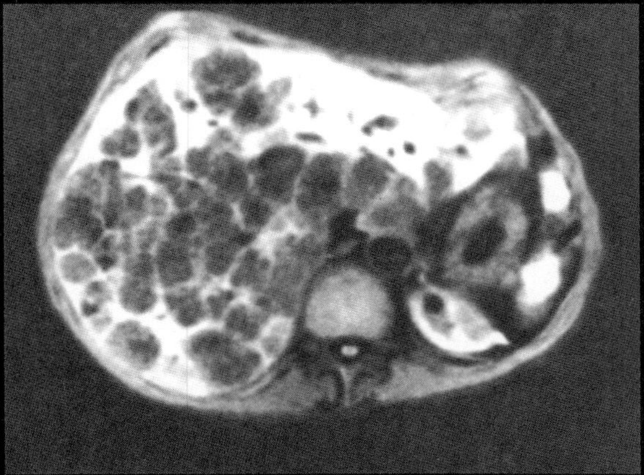

Fig. 9.2 Multiple metastases (courtesy Hammersmith Hospital)

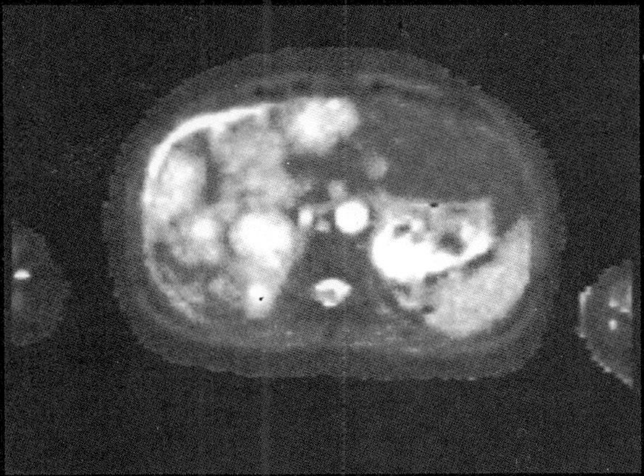

Fig. 9.3 Multiple metastases

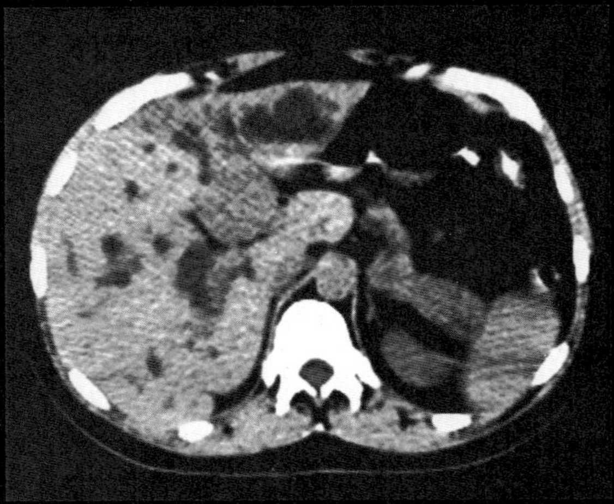

Fig. 9.4 Adenocarcinoma at porta hepatitis; precontrast CT (courtesy Hammersmith Hospital)

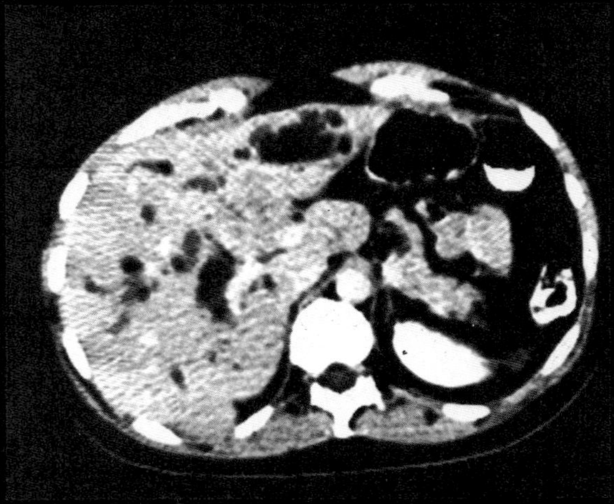

Fig. 9.5 Adenocarcinoma at porta hepatitis; postcontrast CT (courtesy Hammersmith Hospital)

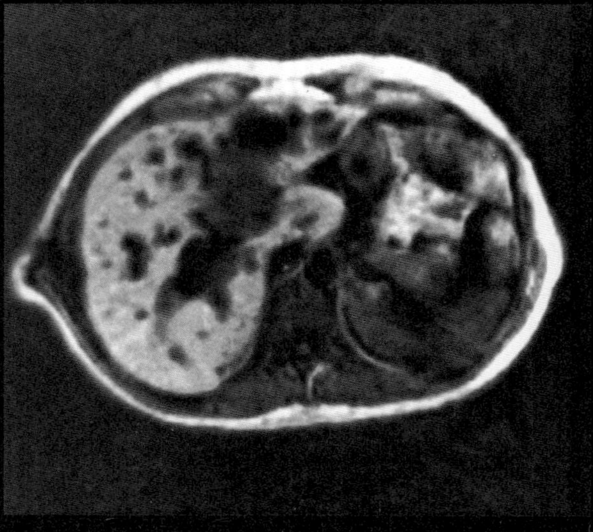

Fig. 9.6 Adenocarcinoma before gadolinium; inversion recovery (courtesy Hammersmith Hospital)

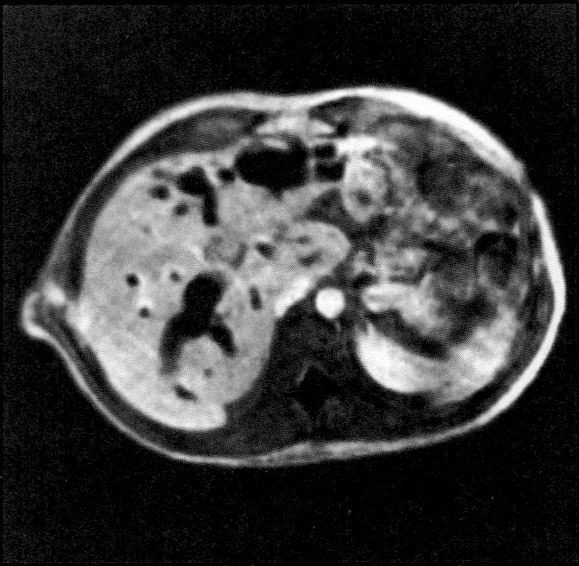

Fig. 9.7 Adenocarcinoma after gadolinium (courtesy Hammersmith Hospital). After gadolinium DTPA the tumour at the porta hepatis enhances but its signal intensity approaches that of liver. Note Higher signal from aorta, IVC and portal veins after gadolinium

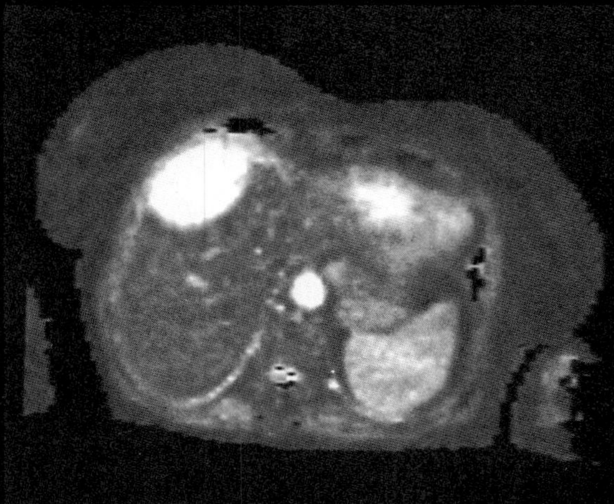

Fig. 9.8 Subphrenic abscess; transverse; calculated T_1

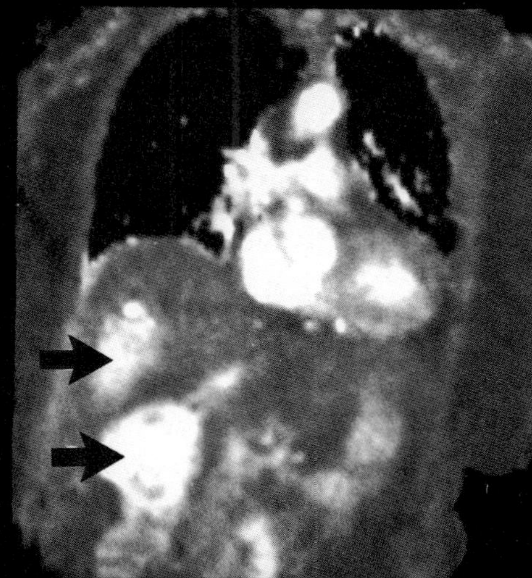

Fig. 9.9 Subphrenic and subhepatic abscess; coronal

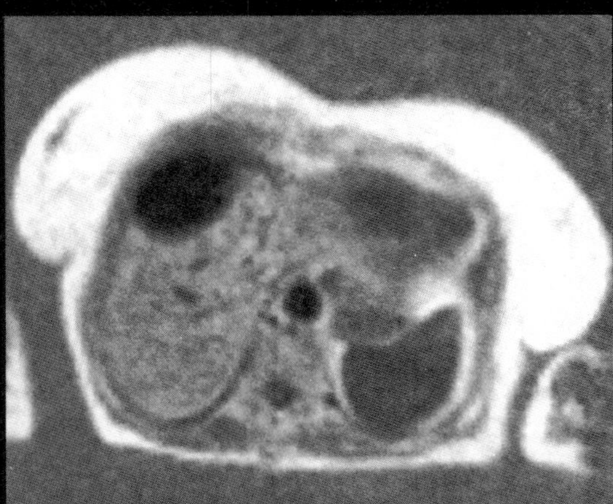

Fig. 9.10 Subphrenic abscess; inversion recovery

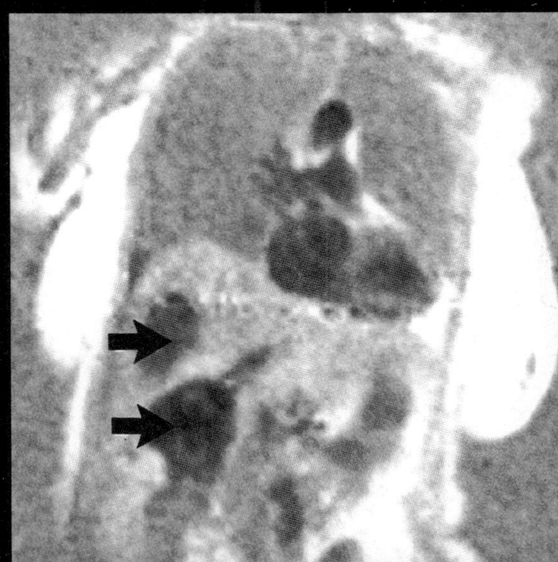

Fig. 9.11 Subphrenic abscess; inversion recovery

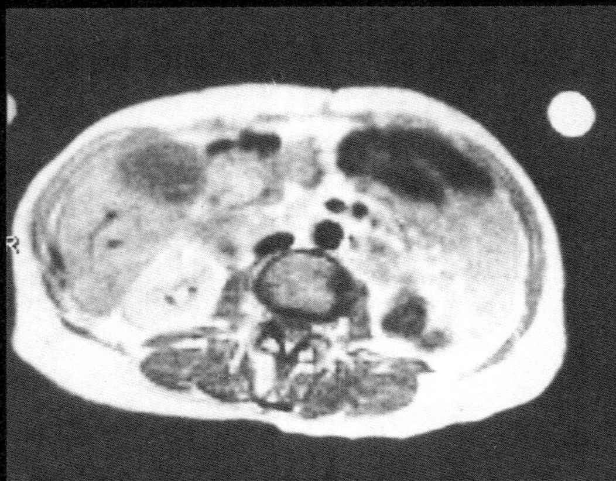

Fig. 9.12 Gallbladder; *TR* 1.5 s, *TE* 28 ms (courtesy UCSF, California)

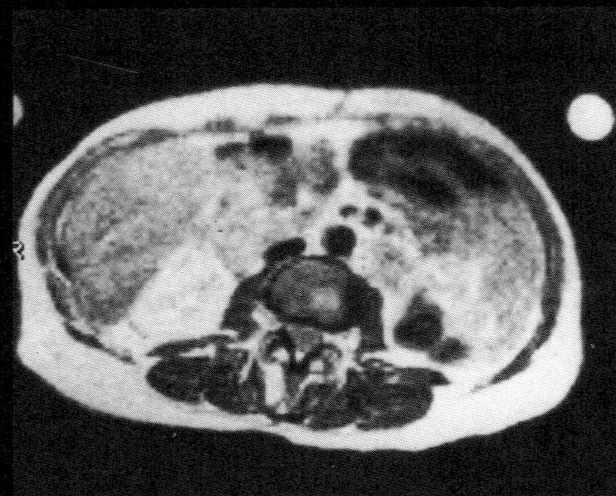

Fig. 9.13 Gallbladder; *TR* 1.5 s, *TE* 56 ms (courtesy UCSF, California)

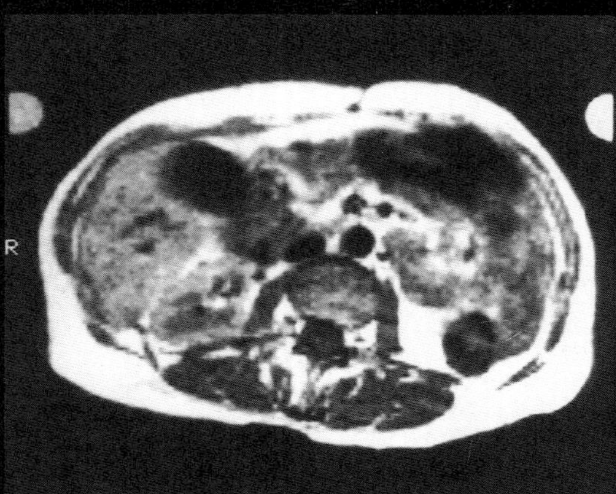

Fig. 9.14 Gallbladder; *TR* 0.5 s, *TE* 28 ms (courtesy UCSF, California)

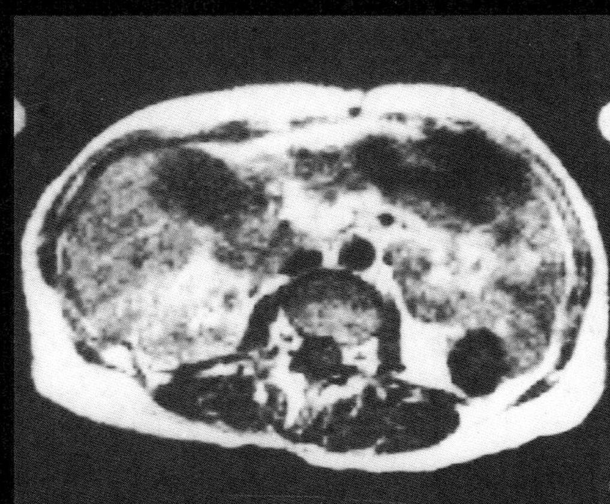

Fig. 9.15 Gallbladder; *TR* 0.5 s, *TE* 56 ms (courtesy UCSF, California)

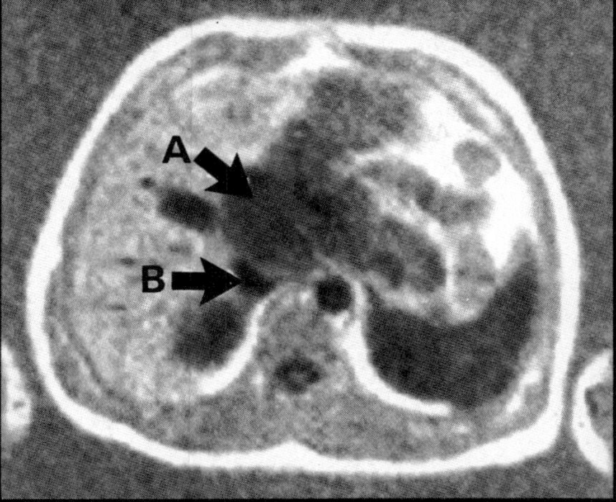

Fig. 9.16 Pancreatic mass; inversion recovery; transverse (A = mass, B = IVC)

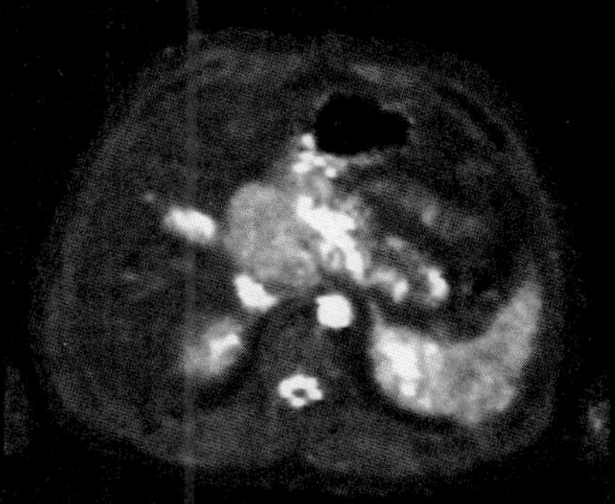

Fig. 9.17 Pancreatic mass; calculated

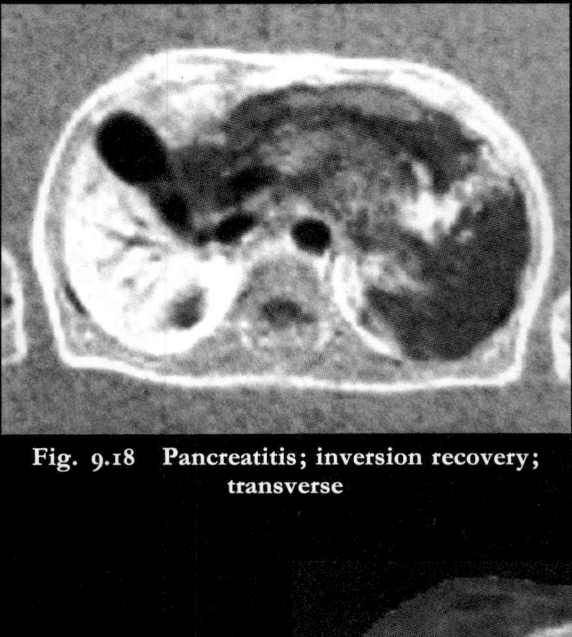

Fig. 9.18 Pancreatitis; inversion recovery; transverse

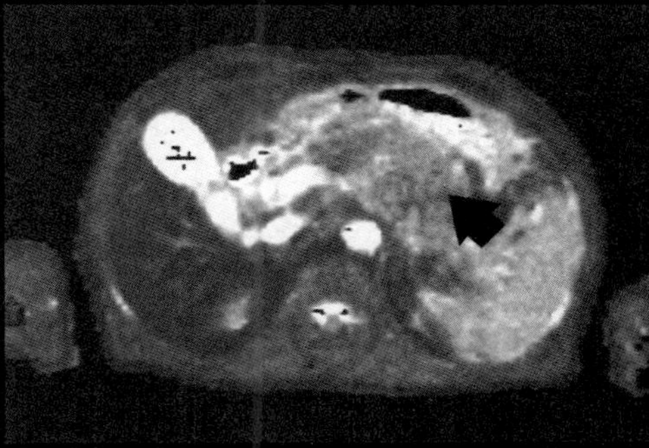

Fig. 9.19 Pancreatitis; calculated T_1

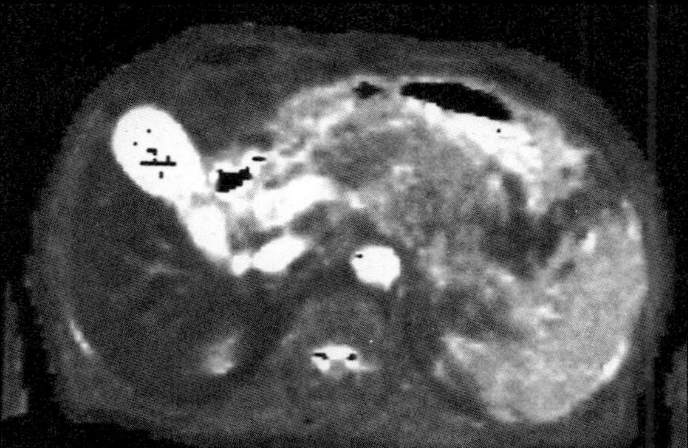

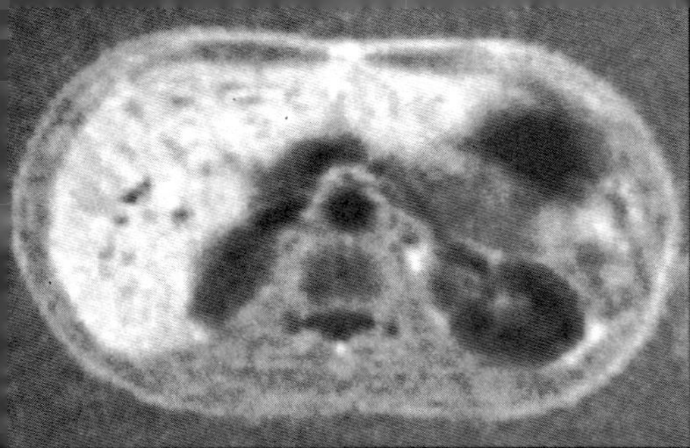

Fig. 9.21 Phaochromocytoma; inversion recovery; transverse. The long T_1 lesion is seen as a region of low MR signal

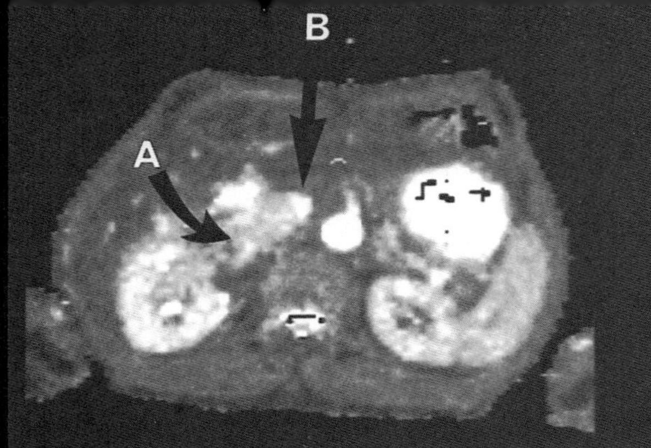

Fig. 9.22 Renal carcinoma extending to the IVC. Calculated T_1 image. (A = Tumour; B = IVC)

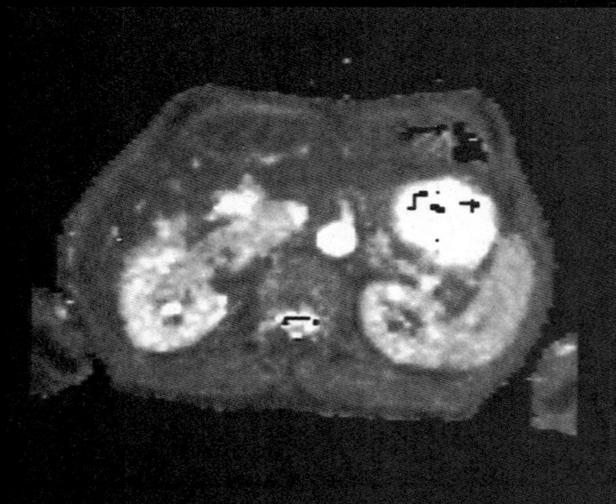

Fig. 9.23 Renal carcinoma extending to the IVC; calculated T_1; transverse

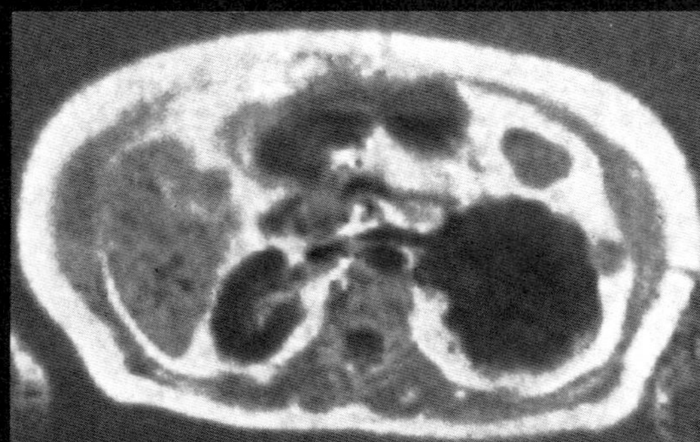

Fig. 9.24 Renal Carcinoma; inversion recovery; transverse

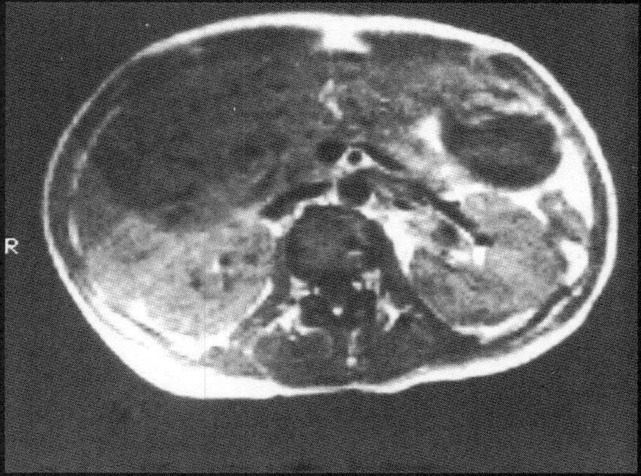

Fig. 9.25 Renal abscess; *TR* 0.5 s, *TE* 28 ms (courtesy UCSF, California)

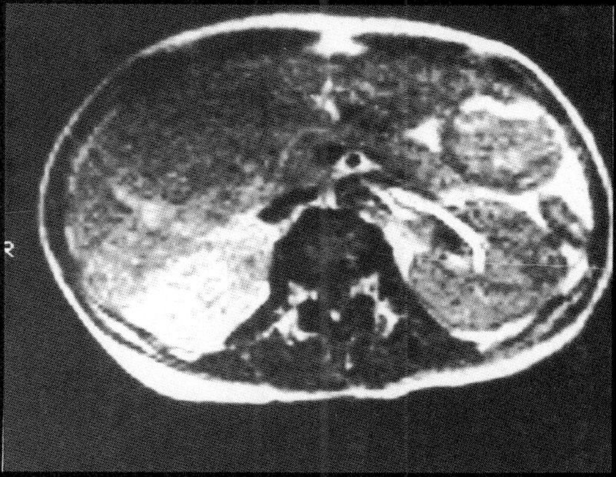

Fig. 9.26 Renal abscess; *TR* 0.5 s, *TE* 56 ms (courtesy UCSF, California)

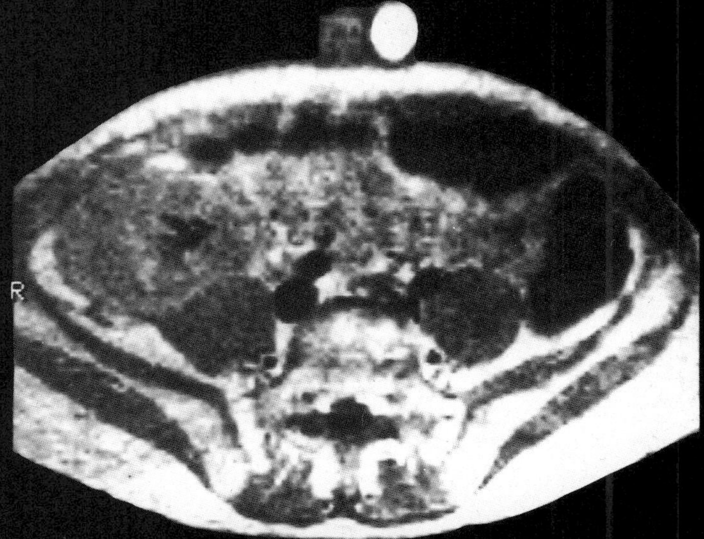

Fig. 9.27 Renal transplant; *TR* 0.5 s, *TE* 28 ms (courtesy UCSF, California)

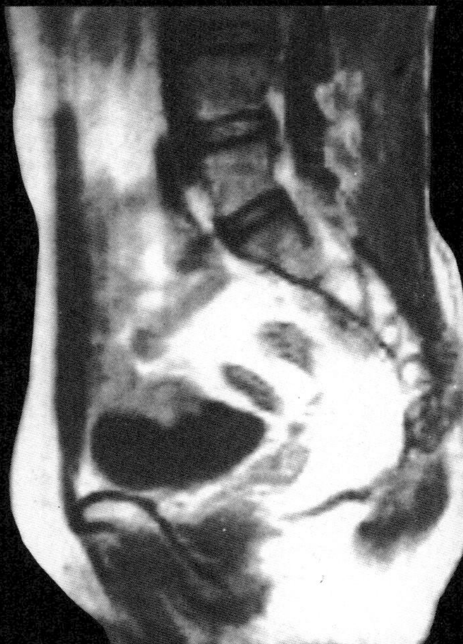

Fig. 9.28 Urachal carcinoma; *TR* 1.5 s, *TE* 28 ms

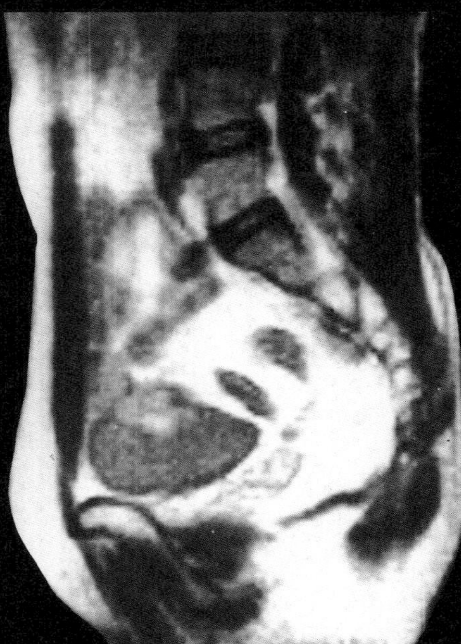

Fig. 9.29 Urachal carcinoma. The lesion on the superior surface of the bladder is seen to give a higher signal on the second echo (56 msec) indicating a prolonged T_2; *TR* 1.5 s, *TE* 56 ms

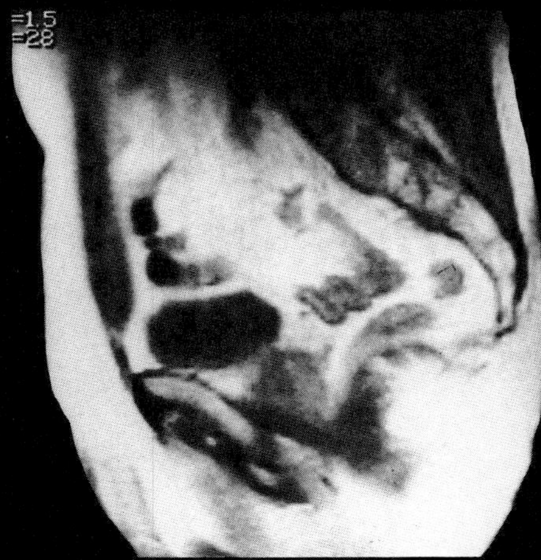

Fig. 9.30 Involvement of seminal vesicles by prostatic carcinoma; *TR* 1.5 s, *TE* 28 ms (courtesy UCSF, California)

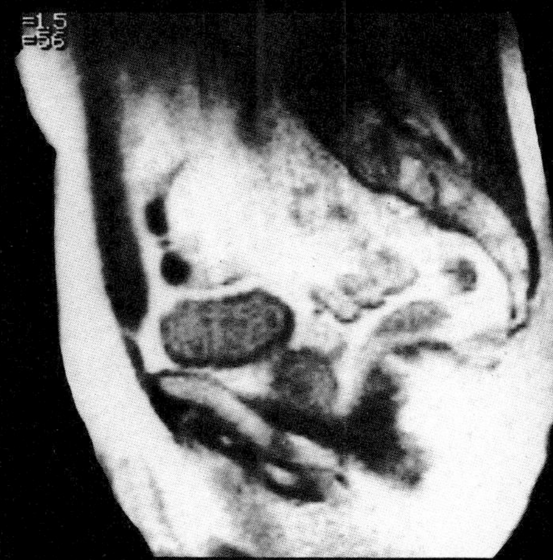

Fig. 9.31 Involvement of seminal vesicles by prostatic carcinoma; *TR* 1.5 s, *TE* 56 ms (courtesy UCSF, California)

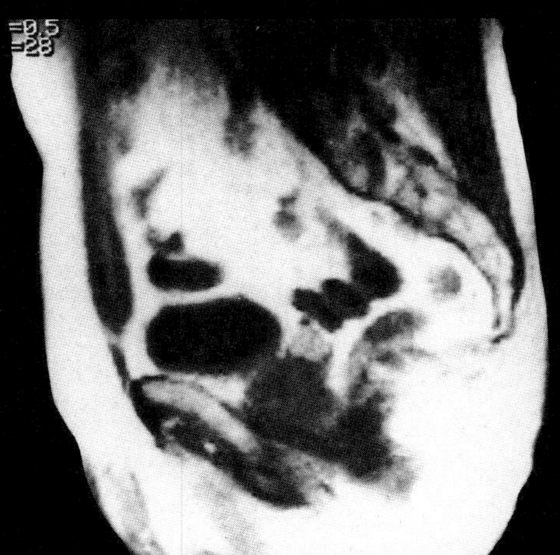

Fig. 9.32 Involvement of seminal vesicles by prostatic carcinoma (courtesy UCSF, California)

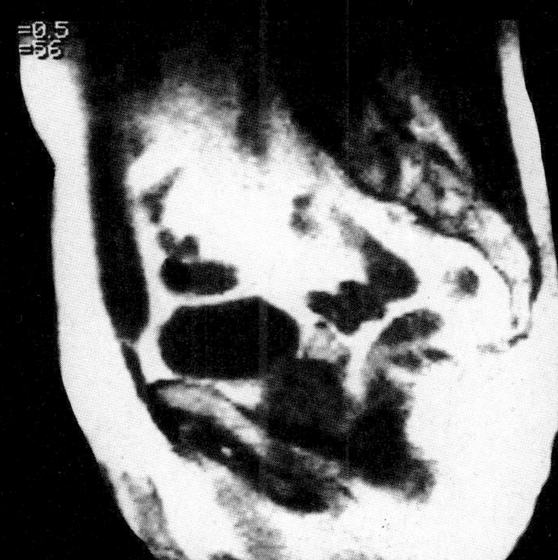

Fig. 9.33 Involvement of seminal vesicles by prostatic carcinoma; *TR* 0.5 s, *TE* 56 ms (courtesy UCSF, California)

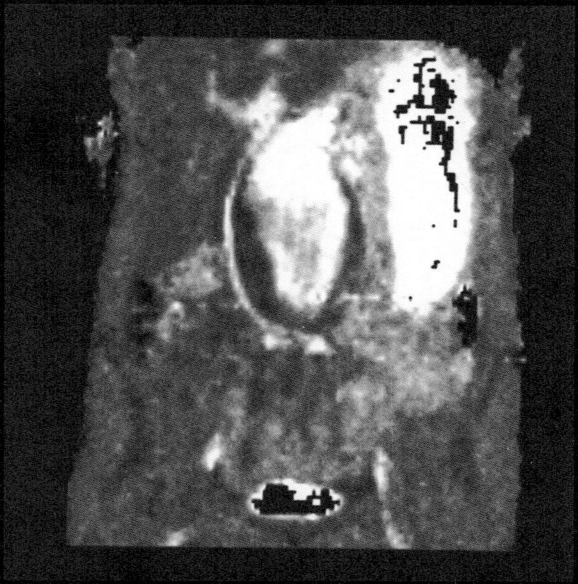

Fig. 9.34 Aortic aneurysm; calculated T_1

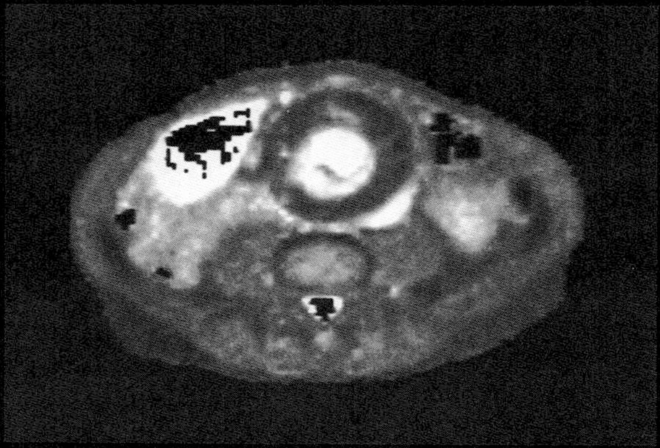

Fig. 9.35 Aortic aneurysm; calculated T_1

10

Imaging the musculoskeletal system

Introduction

Although the major applications of MRI would appear to be in the investigation of pathology within the central nervous system, there is growing evidence that it will also play a major role in the investigation of musculoskeletal disease. This may appear to be contradictory since it has often been stated that MR does not show bone. It is true that MRI does not show the outer thin layer of thin cortical bone, but this only accounts for a very small fraction of any bone. MR does, however, demonstrate the cancellous component of bone very well. Other structures in the musculoskeletal system which can be shown by MR are muscles, ligaments, tendons and blood vessels. The relationship of any pathological lesion to vessels is easily demonstrated without the use of contrast agents and, as in all other areas, the precise location of a lesion can be shown using the multiplanar facility. The increased soft tissue contrast available with MR is another advantage over CT. Metallic objects such as hip prostheses cause a local defect in the MR image due to their effect on the magnetic field, but streaking artefacts do not cause problems, as they do in similar situations in CT. Other structures which give little MR signal are ligaments, but it appears that some signal can be obtained from cartilage as long as the correct pulse sequence is used such as partial saturation recovery sequences with a short TE or inversion recovery sequences with long *TR* and *TI* times (Figs. 10.1 to 10.5—normal imaging).

Neoplastic disease

One of the major applications of MRI in orthopaedics may be in the assessment of primary bone tumours. The choice of pulse sequence is not very critical when trying to define the intramedullary extent of disease since (due to the high fat content) there is considerable contrast between the short T_1 fat in the marrow and the tumour tissue which in almost every instance will have long T_1 values. In the soft tissues, however, it would appear that long *TR*, long *TE* sequences demonstrate the soft tissue involvement best. Thus, by utilising the increased soft tissue contrast, as well as imaging in three planes, the precise extent of neoplasms can be seen. Also their relationships to vessels can be seen without contrast. This is particularly important in cases where conservative surgery is being undertaken, when localisation has to be as precise as possible to allow complete removal of tumour but still leave enough healthy bone for a good cosmetic and functional result. Very precise localisation is also useful in planning fields of radiotherapy treatment. MRI cannot predict the histological type of neoplasm and there is some overlap in the relaxation times of infection and neoplasm. In the investigation of metastatic bone disease isotope bone studies are superior to MRI in the initial detection of disease, and are also cheaper, quicker and more readily obtained. A possible use of MRI might be in a situation where an isotope study is negative but there is strong clinical evidence of secondary bone disease; in this case MRI may be able to exclude or confirm such pathology. Another situation where MRI might be useful is in those patients with degenerative changes which may be responsible for increased isotope uptake. In MRI there will be zero signal from such reactive new bone. MRI will also be useful in defining the local effects of bony secondaries such as pressure and displacement effects in the spine. One other possible use of MRI in neoplastic bone disease is in the follow-up of the condition, as it is thought that changes in relaxation time measurements may be of use in monitoring therapy (Figs. 10.6 to 10.10).

Bone marrow

As well as the changes in the marrow seen in neoplastic conditions MR can also show changes in infection. MR changes have been observed when CT and isotope have both been negative. The contrast between the abnormal and normal marrow is seen best on inversion recovery sequences where normal fatty marrow will be seen as very high signal contrasted with the low signal of infected marrow. Marrow disease most often leads to a replacement of the fat in the marrow by pathological tissue and this replacement of high signal fat usually leads to a reduction in signal intensity. However in aplastic anaemia the marrow fat may actually increase in volume and this may be recognised by a significant increase in MR signal intensity.

Avascular necrosis

This is another area where MRI has been shown to be potentially very useful. Most work has concentrated on the hips, but the findings could be applied to other areas such as the knees. The normal femoral heads are seen as rounded areas of high signal intensity with a central area of slightly lower signal intensity surrounded by a thin rim of compact bone which gives virtually no signal. In cases of avascular necrosis the initial findings are areas of low signal on inversion recovery sequences due to lengthened relaxation times, usually in the superior portion of the head; this may later spread to involve the entire head. It is generally now believed that MRI is superior to other imaging techniques such as CT and isotope studies in the evaluation of avascular necrosis, since, not only does it demonstrate disease in cases where isotope and CT are negative but, due to the multiplanar capability, it can demonstrate the full extent of the process better than these two modalities. The coronal plane is particularly useful when imaging the hips and, coupled with the transverse and/or sagittal planes, allows very precise delineation of the process.

Vertebral column

As in other areas of the body short *TR*, *TE* spin echo sequences are very useful in providing images with an excellent signal-to-noise (S/N) ratio in a relatively short time. This type of sequence can therefore be used initially to provide good anatomical detail. However other pulse sequences which highlight T_1 and T_2 differences are necessary to demonstrate most types of pathology to the maximum advantage, as well as some aspects of normal anatomy. The contrast between tissues is dependent on the relaxation time differences as well as the pulse sequence. With short *TR*, *TE* sequences the signal from CSF will be very low due to its long T_1 and T_2. The contrast between abnormal relaxation time area in the cord and normal cord will also be low on 'short' sequences and 'longer' sequences must be used to accentuate this difference. It must be remembered that, using longer sequences, not only will the signal from the abnormality be increased but that the signal from the immediately adjacent CSF will increase and therefore the *TR* and *TE* must not be increased too much or the abnormality may be obscured by the high signal from the CSF. These very long sequences may, however, be used when contrast between CSF and the disc region is desired; the cord will be totally obscured by the high signal from the CSF but there will be better contrast between the CSF and the low signal of the annulus fibrosus. Immediately within the annulus in the normal situation is the nucleus pulposus. This nucleus becomes dehydrated with age and this causes its relaxation times and proton density to decrease. The value of this is that if a normally hydrated disc is demonstrated it can be confidently stated that the disc has not herniated since all herniated discs are dehydrated. Conversely the presence of a dehydrated disc does not, however, have a direct correlation with clinical symptoms and herniation; many such discs have been observed in asymptomatic patients and volunteers. The presence of a disc herniation will be demonstrated to best effect on long *TR*, *TE* sequences when the extruded disc will be seen as a low intensity structure projecting into the high signal CSF. Deposits of fat occur normally in an epidural location intimately related to the lateral root canals. When these canals become narrowed in lateral root canal stenosis this epidural fat deposit is lost. Although this can be shown by good quality CT, false-negative results may occur. This fat loss can be demonstrated relatively easily by most MR sequences (due to the high signal intensity of fat), particularly when the spine is imaged in a parasagittal plane when comparison can be made with the normal high signal fat above and below the symptomatic level, and in this situation it would appear that the MR abnormality is directly related to pathology as no signal means no fat indicating stenosis.

Disadvantages of MRI of the spine

There are some important disadvantages in MRI of the spine:

(1) Compact bone such as that found in bony lipping and osteophytes cannot be demonstrated unless very large when its presence may be inferred by areas of low signal encroaching on the spinal cord.

(2) The spatial resolution of MRI is inferior to CT. This may be improved with continuing refinement of surface coil and pulse sequences.

Both these drawbacks combine to make MRI a very poor imaging technique at present in the evaluation of acute spinal trauma where small bony fragments pressing on the cord cannot be identified; on the other hand, although the bone may not be visible the resultant displacement of the cord will be easily seen.

This example of spinal trauma also illustrates another important disadvantage of MRI in acute injuries; these patients frequently have multiple injuries requiring fixation with large amounts of metal which may totally exclude them from a high field unit, and even if they can be accommodated may seriously degrade the quality of the image on a lower field system (Figs. 10.11 to 10.17).

Other types of spinal pathology

Syringomyelia

As mentioned in Chapter 7 (p. x) the presence of a syrinx can be easily demonstrated. Short *TR*, *TE* sequences can be used when the signal from the CSF will be low contrasting with the medium signal of the cord. A syrinx can be seen even when the cord is not expanded which may cause false-negative results in CT. The presence of other abnormalities associated with a syrinx such as Arnold Chiari malformation will be readily demonstrated, particularly with the sagittal plane.

Infection

Infection of a disc and the adjacent vertebrae is easily shown by MRI due to the lengthened relaxation times found in infective processes. The nature of the pathology can be inferred from its distribution. Often it will be seen to involve the entire disc space causing loss of differentiation between annulus and nucleus pulposus. The abnormality is best shown by long *TE* sequences and is often observed involving adjacent vertebrae.

Neoplasm

Any neoplastic pathology of the intradural and extradural compartments can be demonstrated relatively easily by MRI. It is a simple matter to separate the pathology from CSF due to the large relaxation time differences present; this can be performed using short *TR*, *TE* sequences but there may be some difficulty in differentiating between tumour and cord. 'Longer' sequences may help to achieve this differentiation.

Vascular malformations

There has been relatively little experience with this type of abnormality and this is limited to cases of arteriovenous malformations. These, in common with other areas of flowing blood, will appear as low signal regions and their nature can be confirmed by employing flow-dependent sequences, for instance saturation recovery with short *TR*. It must be stressed that neither the feeding nor draining vessels can be identified with any degree of confidence and therefore vascular studies are still necessary to obtain this vital information (Fig. 10.18).

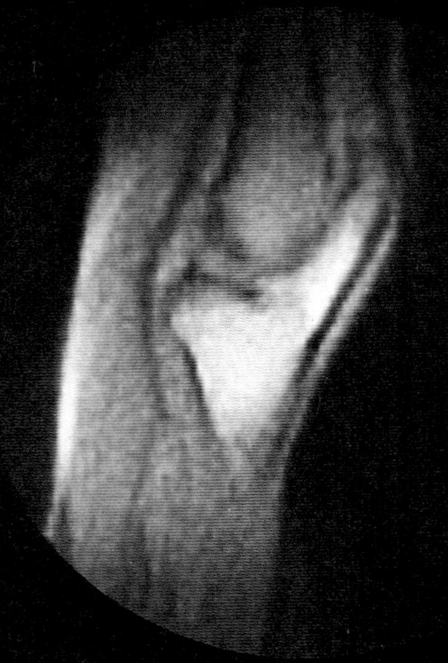

Fig. 10.1 Sagittal knee (courtesy of Queens Medical Centre, Nottingham and *British Journal of Radiology*)

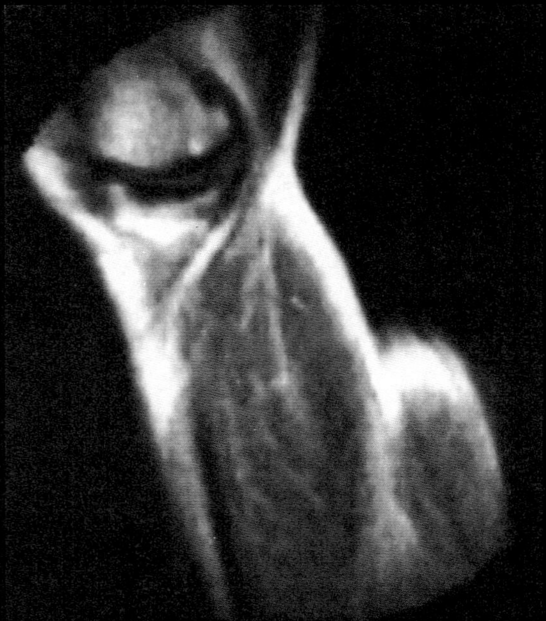

Fig. 10.2 Meniscus (courtesy of Queens Medical Centre, Nottingham and *British Journal of Radiology*)

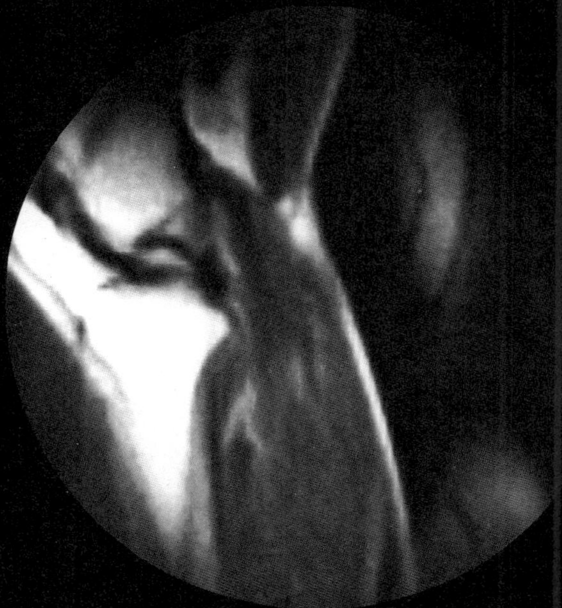

Fig. 10.3 Posterior cruciate (courtesy of Queens Medical Centre, Nottingham and *British Journal of Radiology*)

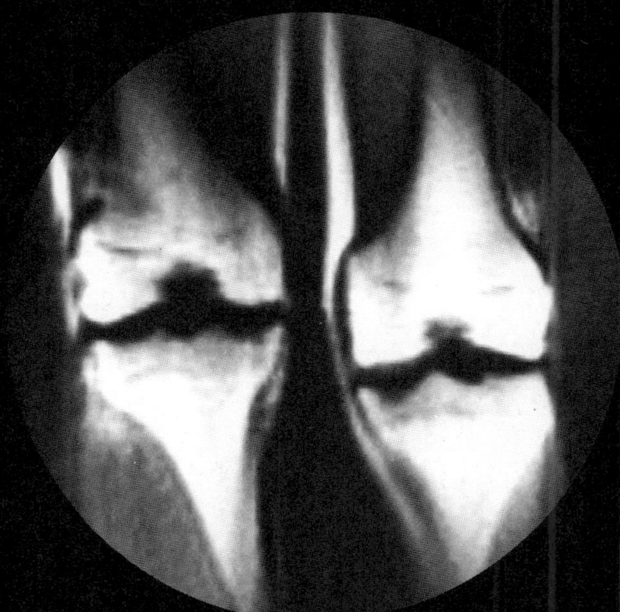

Fig. 10.4 Coronal knee (courtesy of Queens Medical Centre, Nottingham and *British Journal of Radiology*)

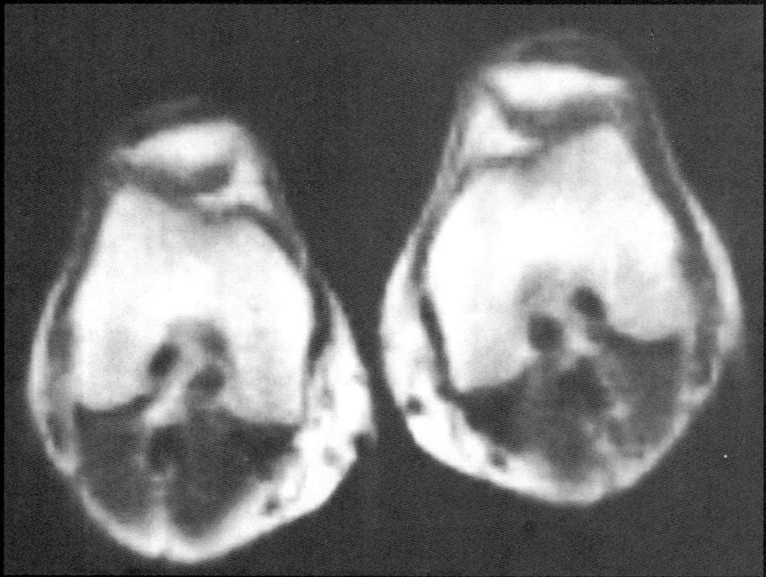

Fig. 10.5 Transverse knee (courtesy of Queens Medical Centre, Nottingham and *British Journal of Radiology*)

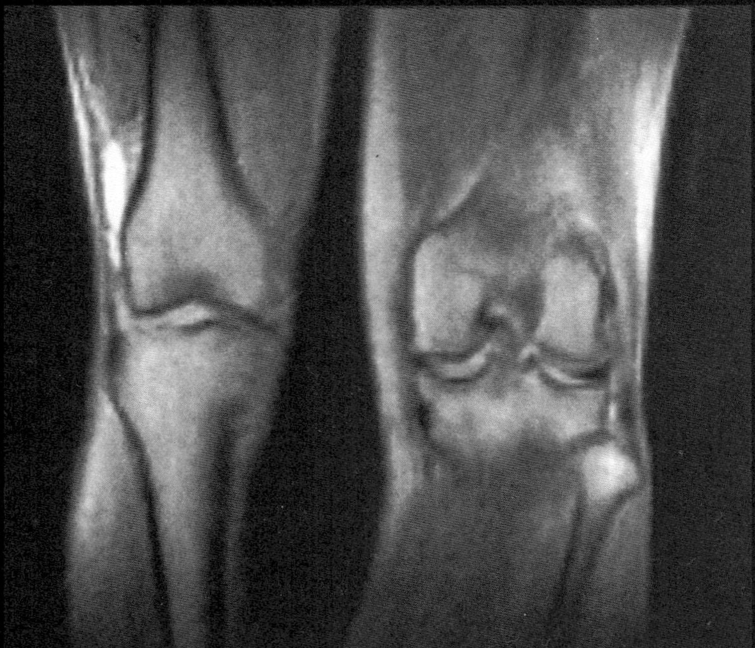

Fig. 10.6 Coronal knees. Cortical bone and the menisci are seen as areas of zero signal on this long *TR*, long *TI* T_1 weighted image. A recent sports injury causing an area of prolonged T_1 is seen adjacent to a lateral femoral condyle

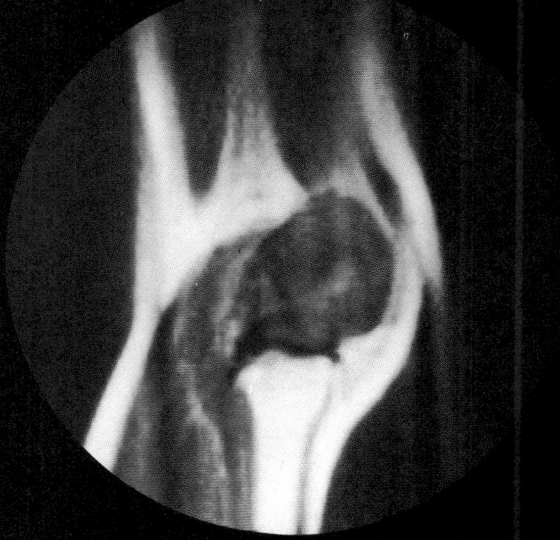

Fig. 10.7 Sagittal osteosarcoma (courtesy of Queens Medical Centre, Nottingham)

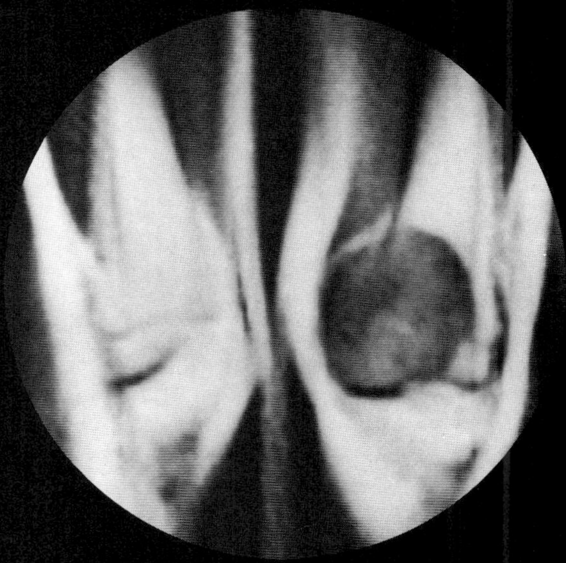

Fig. 10.8 Coronal osteosarcoma (courtesy of Queens Medical Centre, Nottingham). The full extent of the neoplasm is easily seen

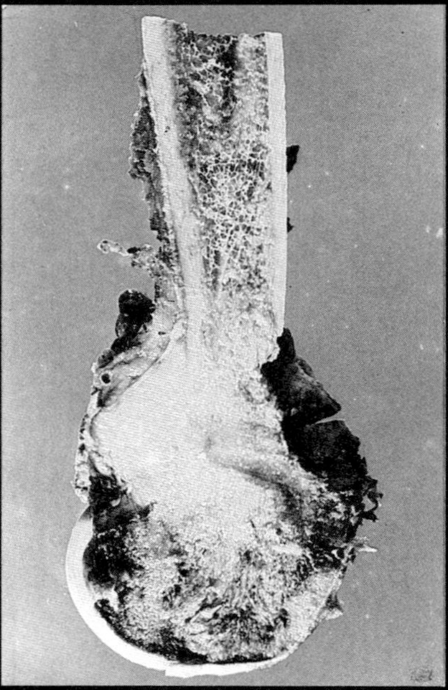

Fig. 10.9 Pathological specimen (courtesy of Queens Medical Centre, Nottingham)

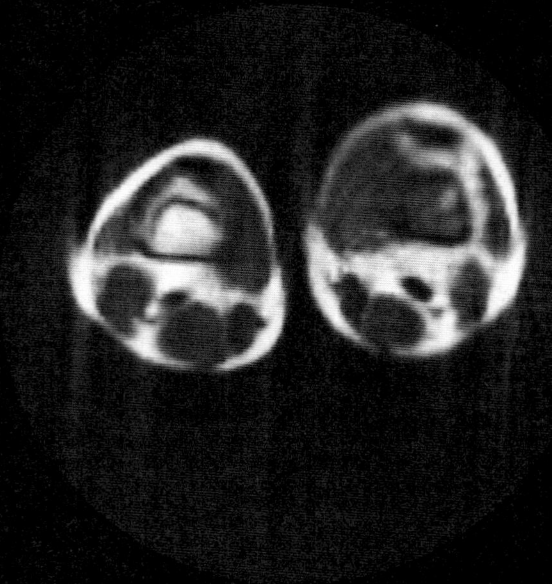

Fig. 10.10 Neoplasm in marrow cavity (courtesy of Queens Medical Centre, Nottingham and *British Journal of Radiology*). Low signal on the abnormal side due to replacement of high signal fat by tumour

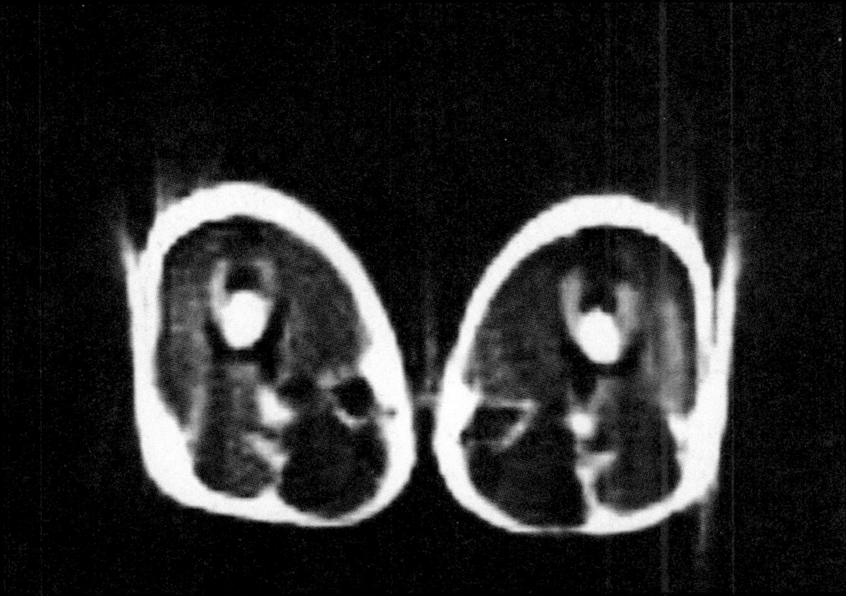

Fig. 10.11 No evidence of tumour in marrow cavity (courtesy of Queens Medical Centre, Nottingham and *British Journal of Radiology*). This image shows high signal from both marrow cavities

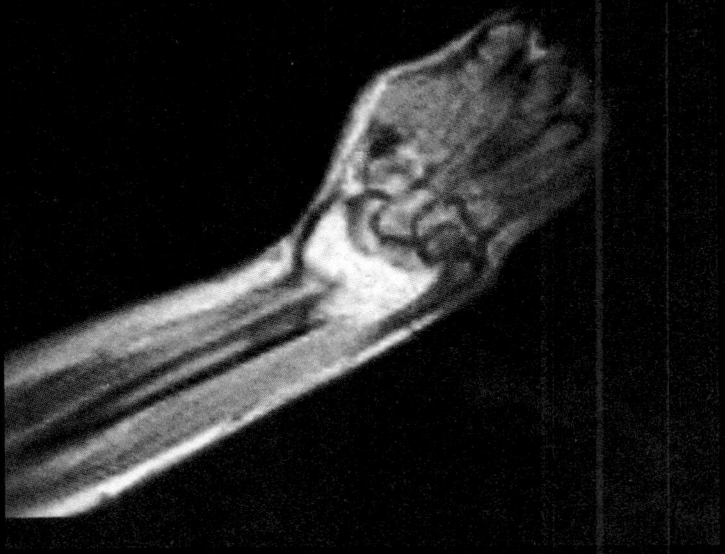

Fig. 10.12 Giant cell tumour. This T_1 weighted image shows a tumour of the distal radius which appears to involve the carpal bones. This involvement was confirmed by surgery

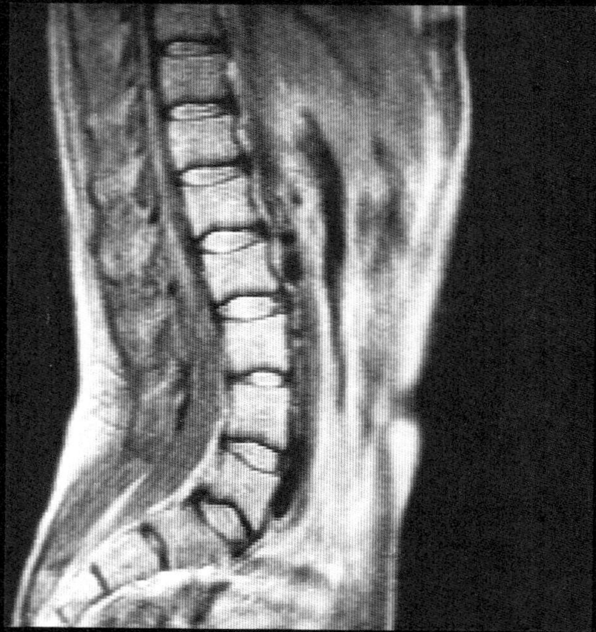

Fig. 10.13 Normal lumbar spine; short *TR* 2 s (courtesy of Cleveland Clinic)

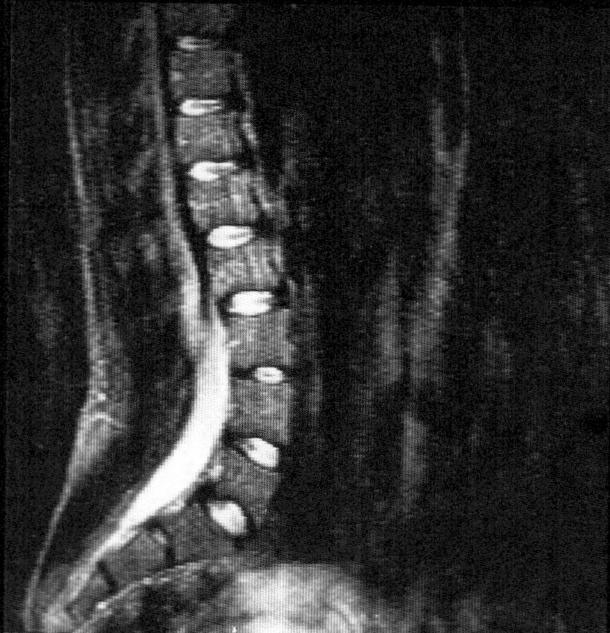

Fig. 10.14 Normal lumbar spine; long *TR* 3 s (courtesy of Cleveland Clinic)

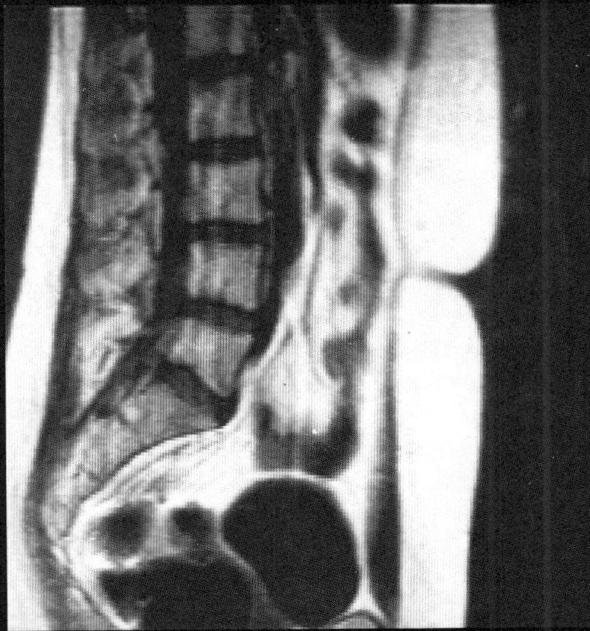

Fig. 10.15 Prolapsed disc; short *TR* 0.2 s, *TE* 30 ms (courtesy of Cleveland Clinic)

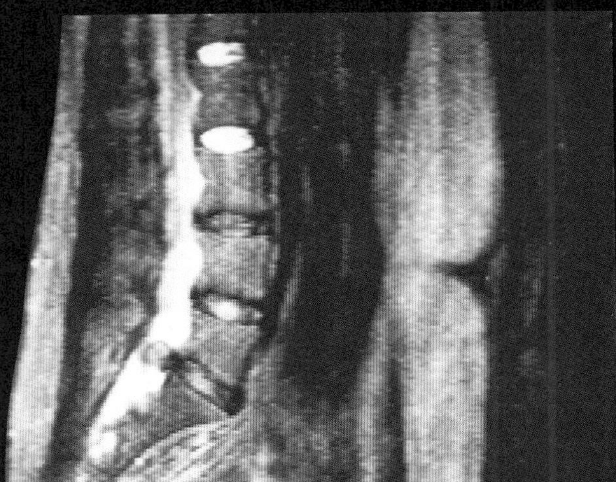

Fig. 10.16 Prolapsed disc; long *TR* 3 s, *TE* 120 ms (courtesy of Cleveland Clinic)

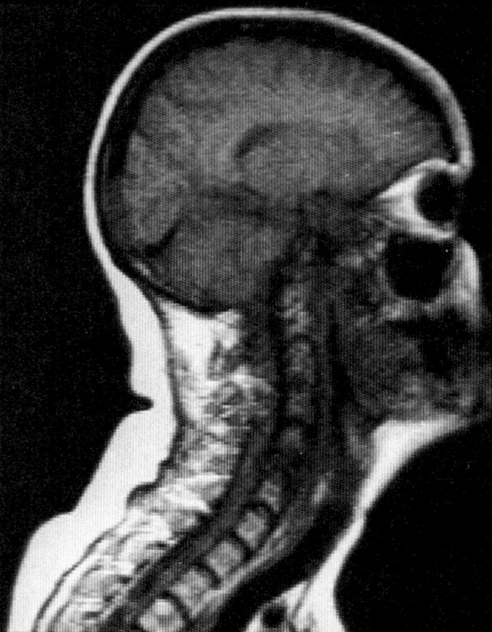

Fig. 10.17 Plasmacytoma C4; short *TR* 0.25 s, *TE* 30 ms (courtesy of Cleveland Clinic)

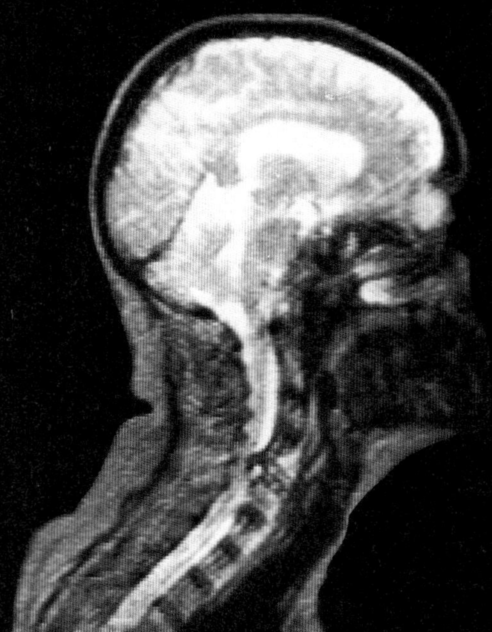

Fig. 10.18 Plasmacytoma C4; long *TR* 3 s, *TE* 120 ms (courtesy of Cleveland Clinic)

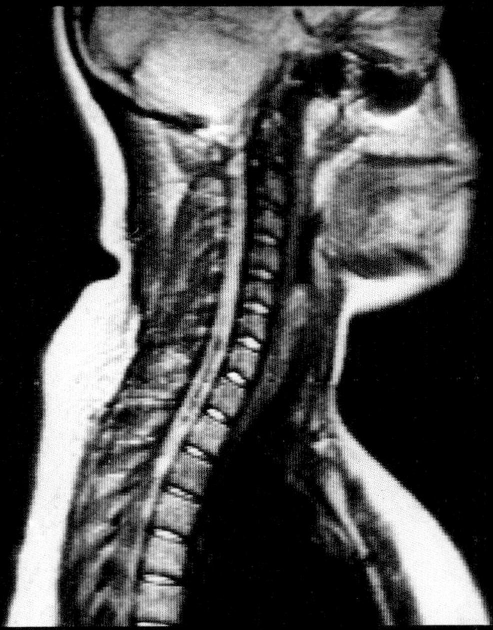

Fig. 10.19 Syrinx; *TR* 0.5 s, *TE* 30 ms (courtesy of Cleveland Clinic)

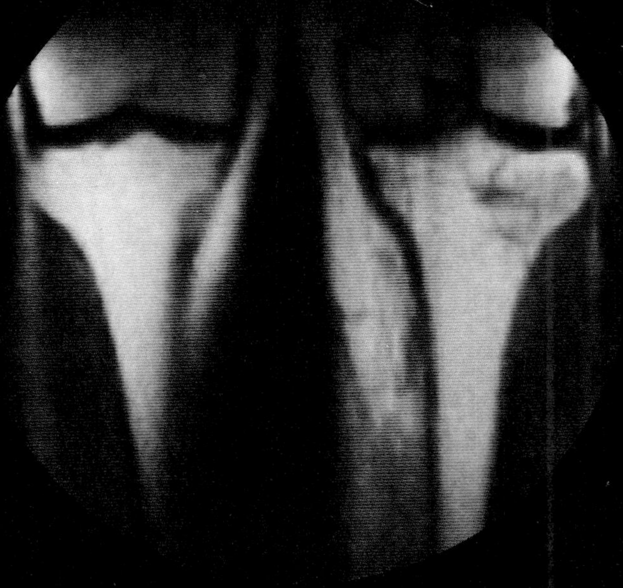

Fig. 10.20 Fracture of tibial spine. (Courtesy of Queens Medical Centre, Nottingham and *British Journal of Radiology*)

References

Bydder G. M., Steiner R. E., Young I. R., Hall A. S., Thomas D. J., Marshall J., Pallis C. A. and Legg N. J. (1982). Clinical NMR imaging of the brain: 140 cases. *Am. J. Radiol;* **139:** 215–236.

Damadian R. (1971). Tumour detection by nuclear magnetic resonance. *Science;* **171:** 1151.

Edelstein W. A., Hutchinson J. M. S., Johnson G. and Redpath T. (1980). Spin-warp NMR imaging and applications to human whole body imaging. *Phys. Med. Biol;* **25:** 751–756.

Gadian D. G. (1980). *Nuclear Magnetic Resonance and its Applications to Living Systems*; Oxford University Press, Oxford.

Hutchinson J. M. S. and Smith, F. W. (1983). NMR clinical results: Aberdeen. In *Nuclear Magnetic Resonance (NMR) Imaging*, eds. Partain C. L., James A. E., Rollo F. D. and Price R. R. W.B. Saunders Co., Philadelphia, USA. pp. 231–249.

Lauterbur P. C. (1973). Image formation by induced local interactions: examples employing nuclear magnetic resonance. *Nature;* **242:** 190–191.

Mansfield P. (1977). Multi-planar image formation using NMR spin echoes. *J. Phys;* (C) **10:** L55–58.

Mansfield P. and Morris P. G. (1982). *NMR Imaging in Biomedicine;* Academic Press, Orlando, USA.

Mathur-De Vré R. (1984). Biomedical implications of the relaxation behaviour of water related to NMR imaging. *Brit. J. Radiol*; **57:** 955–976.

Smith F. W. (1982). Clinical application of NMR tomographic imaging. In *Proceedings of the NMR Symposium, Winston Salem, 1981,* eds. Witcofski R. L., Karstaedt N. and Partain C. L. Bowman Gray School of Medicine Press, pp. 125–132.

Straughan K., Spencer D. H. and Bydder G. M. (1983). NMR clinical results: Hammersmith. In *Nuclear Magnetic Resonance (NMR) Imaging;* eds. Partain C. L., James A. E., Rollo F. D. and Price R. R. W. B. Saunders Co., Philadelphia, USA. pp. 195–206.

Wehrli F. W., MacFall J. R., Shutts D., Breger R. and Herfkens R. J. (1984). Mechanisms of contrast in NMR imaging. *J. Comput. Assist. Tomogr;* **8:** 369–380.

Selected References

Head and Neck

Bradley W. G., Waluch V., Brant-Zawadski M. and Wycoff R. R. (1984). Patchy periventricular white matter lesions in the elderly: A common observation during NMR imaging. *Non-invasive Imaging;* **1:** 35–42.

Brant-Zawadski M., Davis P. L., Crooks L. E., Mills C. M., Norman D., Newton T. H., Sheldon P. and Kaufmann L. (1983). NMR demonstration of cerebral abnormalities: Comparison with CT. *Am. J. Roent;* **140:** 847–54.

Bydder G. M., Steiner R. E. (1982). NMR imaging of the brain. *Neuroradiology;* **23:** 147–57.

Bydder G. M., Steiner R. E., Thomas D. J., Marshall J., Gillerdale D. J. and Young I. R. (1983). NMR imaging of the posterior fossa in 50 cases. *Clin. Radiol;* **34:** 173–88.

Bydder G. M., Steiner R. E., Young I. R., Hall A. S., Thomas D. J., Marshall J., Pallis C. A. and Legg N. J. (1982). Clinical NMR imaging of the brain: 140 cases. *Am. J. Roent;* **139:** 215–36.

Carr D. H., Brown J., Bydder G. M., Weinemann H. J., Speck U., Thomas D. J. and Young I. R. Clinical use of intravenous gadolinium–DTPA as a contrast agent in NMR imaging of cerebral tumours. *Lancet;* **1:** 484–86.

Hans J. S., Benson J., Bonstelle C. *et al.* (1984). Magnetic resonance imaging of the orbit: A preliminary experience. *Radiology;* **150:** 755.

Hawkes R. C., Holland G. N., Moore W. S. and Worthington B. S. (1980). Nuclear magnetic resonance (NMR) tomography of the brain: A preliminary clinical assessment with demonstration of pathology. *J. Comput. Assist. Tomogr;* **4:** 577–86.

Holland G. N., Hawkes R. C., Moore and Moore W. S. (1980). Nuclear magnetic resonance (NMR) tomography of the brain: Coronal and sagittal sections. *J. Comput. Assist. Tomogr;* **4:** 429–33.

Johnson M. A., Pennock J. M., Bydder G. M., Steiner R. E., Thomas D. J., Hayward R., Bryant D. R. T., Payne J. A., Levine M. L., Whitelaw A., Dubowitz L. M. S. and Dubowitz V. (1983). Clinical NMR imaging of the brain in children: Normal and neurological disease. *Am.J. Neuroradiol;* **4:** 1013–26 and *Am. J. Roent;* **141:** 1005–18.

Lawler G. A., Pennock J. M., Steiner R. E., Jenkins W. J., Sherlock S. and Young I. R. (1983). NMR imaging in Wilson's disease. *J. Comput. Assist. Tomogr;* **7:** 1–8.

Randell C. P., Collins A. G., Hayward R., Thomas D. J., McDonnell M. J., Orr J. S., Bydder G. M. and Steiner R. E. (1983). Nuclear magnetic resonance imaging of the posterior fossa tumours. *Am. J. Roent;* **141:** 489–96.

Sipponen J. T., Kasle M., Ketonen L., Sepponen R. E., Katevuok K. and Suvula A. (1983). Serial nuclear magnetic resonance (NMR) in patients with cerebral infarction. *J. Comput. Assist. Tomogr;* **7:** 585–89.

Sipponen J. T., Sepponen R. E. and Suvula A. (1984). Chronic subdural haematoma demonstration by magnetic resonance. *Radiology;* **150:** 79–85.

Sipponen J. T., Sepponen R. E. and Suvula A. (1983). Nuclear magnetic resonance (NMR) imaging of intracranial haemorrhage in the acute and resolving phases. *J. Comput. Assist. Tomogr;* **7:** 954–59.

Tsutoma A., Tamon I., Hirokazu S. *et al.* (1984). Magnetic resonance imaging of brain tumors: measurements of T_1. *Radiology;* **150:** 95.

Worthington B. S., Kean D. M., Hawkes R. C., Holland G. N., Moore W. S. and Corstan R. (1983). Nuclear magnetic resonance imaging in recognition of giant intracranial aneurysms. *Am. J. Neuroradiol;* **4:** 836–36.

Young I. R., Hall A. S., Pallis C. A., Legg N. J., Bydder G. M. and Steiner R. E. (1983). Nuclear magnetic imaging in white matter disease of the brain using spin echo sequences. *J. Comput. Assist. Tomogr;* **7:** 290–94.

Abdomen

Borkowski G. P., Buonocore E., George C. *et al.* (1983). NMR imaging in the evaluation of the liver: A preliminary experience. *J. Comput. Assist. Tomogr;* **7:** 768.

Bryan P. J., Butler H. E., LiPuma J. P. *et al.* (1983). NMR scanning of the pelvis: Initial experience with a 0.3T system. *Am. J. Roent;* **141:** 1111–18.

Crooks L. E. *et al.* (1983). NMR imaging of the adrenal gland: A preliminary report. *Radiology;* **147:** 55.

Hawkes R. C., Holland G. S., Moore W. S. *et al.* (1981). NMR tomography of the normal abdomen. *J. Comput. Assist. Tomogr;* **5:** 613.

Hricak H., Alper C., Crooks L. E. and Sheldon P. E. (1983). Magnetic resonance imaging of the female pelvis: Initial experience. *Am. J. Roent;* **141:** 1119–28.

Hricak H., Crooks L., Sheldon P. and Kaufmann L. (1983). Nuclear magnetic resonance imaging of the kidney. *Radiology;* **146:** 425–32.

Hricak H., Fily R. A., Margulis A. R. *et al.* (1983). Work in progress. NMR Imaging of the gall-bladder. *Radiology*; **147**: 155.

Hricak H., Williams R. D., Moon K. L., Moss A. A., Alpers C., Crooks L. E. and Kaufmann L. (1983). Nuclear magnetic resonance imaging of the kidney: Renal masses. *Radiology;* **147**: 765–72.

Hricak H., Williams R. D., Spring D. B. *et al.* (1983). Anatomy and pathology of the male pelvis by magnetic resonance imaging. *Am. J. Roent;* **141**: 1101–10.

Leung A. W. L., Bydder G. M., Steiner R. E. *et al.* (1984). MRI of the kidneys. *Am. J. Roent;* **143**: 1215.

London D. A., Davis P. L., Williams R. D., Crooks L. E., Sheldon P. E. and Gooding C. A. (1983). Nuclear magnetic resonance imaging of induced renal lesions. *Radiology;* **148**: 167–73.

Moss A. A., Goldberg H., Stark D. *et al.* (1984). Hepatic tumours: Magnetic resonance and CT appearance. *Radiology;* **150**: 141.

Rosen B., Carter E., Pykett I. *et al.* (1985). Proton chemical shift imaging: An evaluation of its clinical potential using an in vivo fatty liver model. *Radiology;* **154**: 469.

Smith F. W. Mallard J. R., Reid A., Hutchinson J. M. S. (1982). NMR imaging of the pancreas. *Radiology;* **142**: 677.

Smith F. W., Mallard J. R., Reid A., Hutchinson J. M. S. (1981). NMR imaging of the liver: Initial experience, NMR tomographic imaging in liver disease. *Lancet;* **I**: 963.

Stark D. D., Goldberg H., Moss A., Bass N. (1984). Chronic liver disease: Evaluation by magnetic resonance. *Radiology;* **150**: 149.

Stark D. D., Moss A., Goldberg H. *et al.* (1984). Magnetic resonance and CT of the normal and diseased pancreas: A comparative study. *Radiology;* **150**: 153.

Stark D. D., Bass N., Moss A. *et al.* (1983). NMR imaging of experimentally induced liver disease. *Radiology;* **148**: 743.

Thorax

Alfidi R. J., Haaga J. R., Yousef S. J. *et al.* (1982). Preliminary experimental results in humans and animals with superconducting whole body nuclear magnetic resonance scanner. *Radiology;* **143**: 175–81.

Brady T. J., Goldman M. R., Hinshaw W. S. *et al.* (1982). Nuclear magnetic resonance imaging for high resolution delineation of myocardial infarction using paramagnetic enhancement of proton signal. *Radiology;* **144**: 343–47.

El Yousef S. J., Duchesneau R., Alfidi R. J. *et al.* (1984). Magnetic resonance imaging of the breast. *Radiology;* **150**: 761.

Fletcher B. D., Jacobstein M. D., Nelson A. D. *et al.* (1984). Gated magnetic resonance imaging of congenital cardiac malformations. *Radiology;* **150**: 137–40.

Gamsu G., Webb W. R., Sheldon P. *et al.* (1983). Nuclear magnetic resonance imaging of the thorax. *Radiology;* **147**: 473–80.

Herfkens R. J., Higgins C. B., Hricak H. *et al.* (1983). Nuclear magnetic resonance imaging of the cardiovascular system: Normal and pathological findings. *Radiology;* **147**: 749–59.

Higgins C. B., Herfkens R., Lipton M. J. *et al.* (1983). Nuclear magnetic resonance of acute myocardial infarction in dogs: Alterations in magnetic relaxation times. *Am. J. Cardiol;* **52**: 184–88.

Higgins C. B., Lanzer P., Stark D. *et al.* (1984). Imaging by nuclear magnetic resonance in patients with chronic ischaemic heart disease. *Circulation;* **69**: 523–31.

Kaufmann L., Crooks L. E., Sheldon P. *et al.* (1983). The potential impact of nuclear magnetic resonance imaging on cardiovascular diagnosis. *Circulation;* **67:** 251–57.

Lanzer P., Botvinick E. H., Schiller N. B. *et al.* (1984). Cardiac imaging using gated magnetic resonance. *Radiology;* **150:** 121–27.

New P. J. F., Rosen B. R., Brady T. *et al.* (1983). Potential hazards and artifacts of ferromagnetic surgical and dental materials and devices in nuclear magnetic resonance imaging. *Radiology;* **147:** 139–48.

O'Donovan P. B., Ross J., Sivak E. *et al.* (1984). Pictorial essay: MRI of the thorax: The advantages of sagittal and coronal planes. *Am. J. Roent;* **143:** 1211.

Pavlicek W., Geisinger M., Castle L. *et al.* (1983). The effects of nuclear magnetic resonance on patients with cardiac pacemakers. *Radiology;* **147:** 149–53.

Wesbey G., Higgins C. B. *et al.* (1984). Imaging and characterisation of acute myocardial infarction in vivo by gated nuclear magnetic resonance. *Circulation;* **69:**125–30.

Orthopaedics

Kean D. M., Worthington B. S., Preston B. J. *et al.* (1983). Nuclear magnetic resonance imaging of the knee: Examples of normal anatomy and pathology. *Brit. J. Radiol;* **56:** 355–64.

Kean D. M., Worthington B. S., Hawkes R. C. *et al.* (1984). Role of NMR in evaluation of musculoskeletal disease. *Applied Radiology,* **13:** 102–8.

Modic M. T., Weinstein M. A., Pavlicek W. *et al.* (1983). Magnetic resonance of the cervical spine: Clinical and pulse techniques considerations. *Am. J. Roent;* **141:** 1129–36.

Modic M. T., Weinstein M. A., Pavlicek W. *et al.* (1983). NMR of the spine. *Radiology;* **148:** 757–62.

Moon K. L., Genant H. K., Helms C. A. *et al.* (1983). Musculoskeletal applications of NMR. *Radiology;* **147:** 161–71.

Totty W. G., Murphy W. A., Ganz W. *et al.* (1984). MRI of the normal and ischaemic femoral head. *Am. J. Roent;* **143:** 1273.

Index